African Traditional Religion Encounters Christianity

African Traditional Religion Encounters Christianity

The Resilience of a Demonized Religion

John Chitakure

◆PICKWICK *Publications* • Eugene, Oregon

AFRICAN TRADITIONAL RELIGION ENCOUNTERS CHRISTIANITY
The Resilience of a Demonized Religion

Copyright © 2017 John Chitakure. All rights reserved. Except for brief quotations in critical publications or reviews, no part of this book may be reproduced in any manner without prior written permission from the publisher. Write: Permissions, Wipf and Stock Publishers, 199 W. 8th Ave., Suite 3, Eugene, OR 97401.

Pickwick Publications
An Imprint of Wipf and Stock Publishers
199 W. 8th Ave., Suite 3
Eugene, OR 97401

www.wipfandstock.com

PAPERBACK ISBN: 978-1-5326-1854-3
HARDCOVER ISBN: 978-1-4982-4420-6
EBOOK ISBN: 978-1-4982-4419-0

Cataloguing-in-Publication data:

Names: Chitakure, John.

Title: African traditional religion encounters Christianity : the resilience of a demonized religion / John Chitakure.

Description: Eugene, OR: Pickwick Publications, 2017 | Includes bibliographical references and index.

Identifiers: ISBN 978-1-5326-1854-3 (paperback) | ISBN 978-1-4982-4420-6 (hardcover) | ISBN 978-1-4982-4419-0 (ebook)

Subjects: LCSH: Christianity—Africa, Sub-Saharan | Africa, Sub-Saharan—Religion | Africa, Sub-Saharan—Religious life and customs | Theology, Doctrinal—Africa, Sub-Saharan | Medicine, African Traditional | Witchcraft | Ancestor worship | Zimbabwe—Church history

Classification: BR1430 C45 2017 (print) | BR1430 (ebook)

Manufactured in the U.S.A.   10/25/17

To all the Christian missionaries, for their zeal, commitment, and tenacity, and to my *mbuya* (grandmother's sister) Mai Zhezha Chineni Mashanda Mutinha, aka VaChipembere—a traditional medical practitioner, who pursued her calling until she joined the ancestors.

USA Student: Professor, why do you always share African stories with us? Why don't you tell us American stories?

Professor: Thank you student, for your honest observation and questions. I do it for three reasons. First, you already know American stories, and I don't want to repeat them. Second, I am African, and I don't know many American stories. Third, I do it to enrich your worldviews. Since you already know American stories, I shall tell you African stories, and in the end, you will have two sets of stories—one American and the other African. That combination will give you two perspectives from which to understand and interpret phenomena. The possession of more than one view makes you richer, smarter, and more diversified than any other American student that has never been taught by an African professor.

Contents

Map of Zimbabwe: Provinces | viii
Map of Africa | ix

Preface | xi
Acknowledgements | xiii
Abbreviations | xiv

Introduction | 1
1. Christianity Comes to Zimbabwe | 11
2. Rites of Passage | 31
3. The Shona Concept of God | 69
4. The Centrality of Ancestors | 79
5. Avenging Spirits | 99
6. Witchcraft | 115
7. Alien Spirits | 140
8. Traditional Medical Practitioners | 148
9. African Independent Churches | 163
10. Women in African Traditional Religion | 186
11. Shona Ethics | 199

Bibliography | 215
Index | 219

Map of Zimbabwe: Provinces

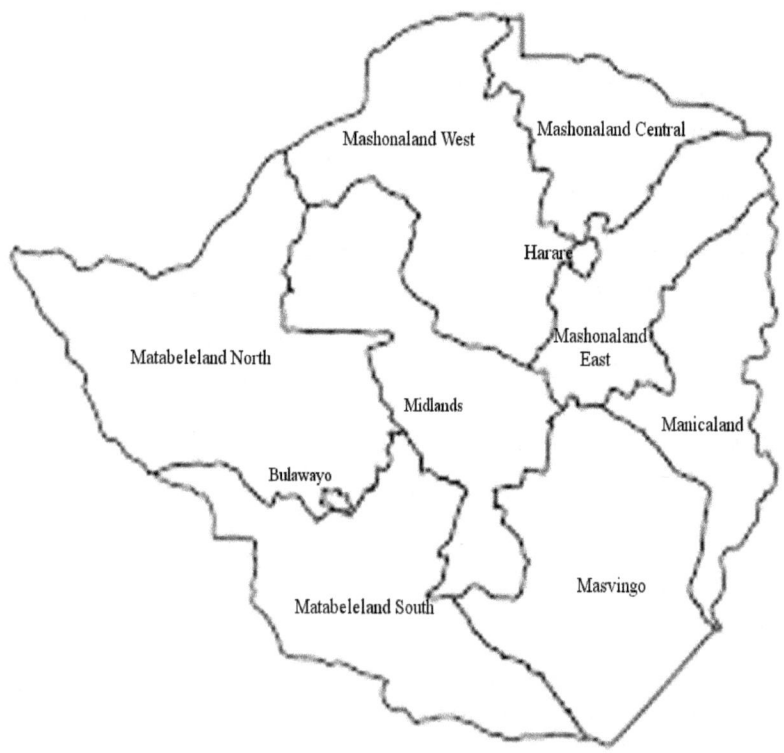

Map created by Nyasha Theobald Chitakure

This map has been adapted from John Chitakure, *Shona Women in Zimbabwe—A Purchased People?* AFRICS (Eugene, OR: Pickwick, 2016).

Map of Africa

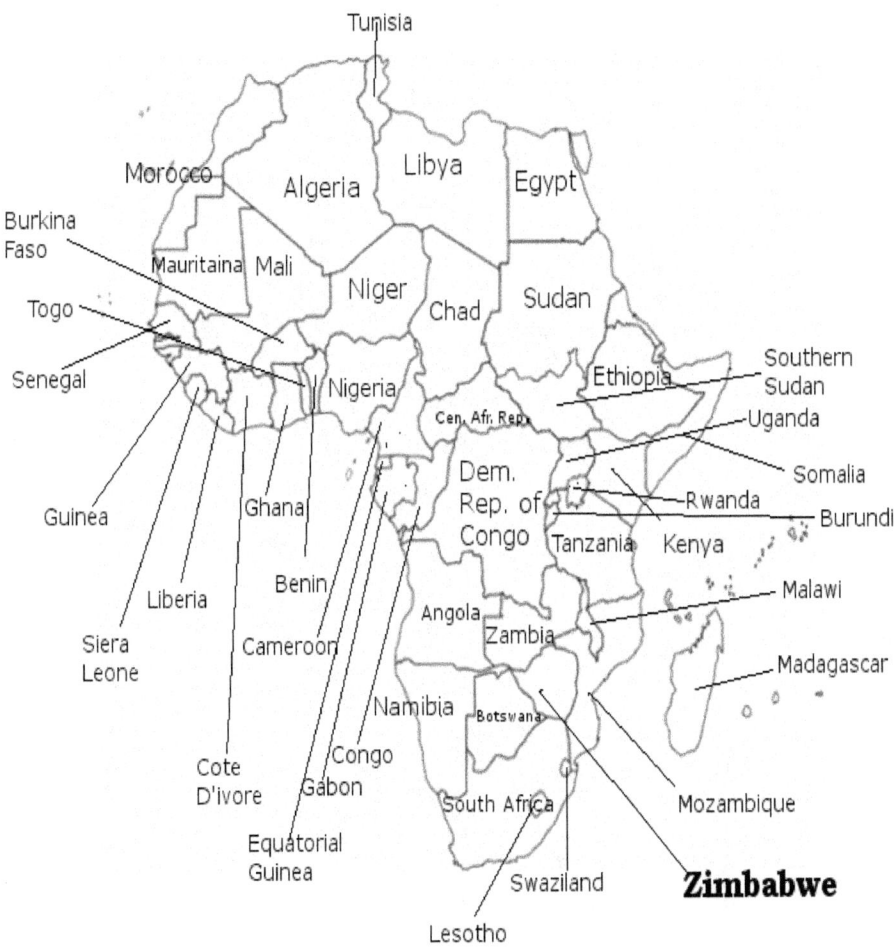

Map created by Mufaro Sean Chitakure

This map has been adapted from John Chitakure, *Shona Women in Zimbabwe—A Purchased People?* AFRICS (Eugene, OR: Pickwick, 2016).

Preface

Most scholars of African Traditional Religion concur that it is impossible to write about Africans and their religions as a homogenous group, despite the many commonalities that most of them share. There are fifty-four countries in Africa, each consisting of several hundreds of ethnic groups. Some estimates say that Africa is home to over three thousand different ethnic groups, and its people speak over two thousand indigenous languages. Zimbabwe alone is home to over ten different ethnic groups, each with its own cultural variations. Zimbabwe is home to the Karanga, Zezuru, Korekore, Ndau, Manyika, Shangani, Kalanga, Nambya, Ndebele, Venda, Tonga, and Whites, among others. The cultural diversity that is found in Africa and each particular country has led some scholars to argue that one can only talk of African Traditional Religions in the plural, not in the singular. However, other researchers have advocated for a singular traditional religion because of the many similarities among the people of Africa.

This book does not claim to speak for all Africans, although it does not shy away from making general references to the shared experiences of the African peoples. Although this book is written from the perspective of the Shona people of Zimbabwe, most of the topics that it explores are common to the African people. Topics such as ancestors, witchcraft, God, rites of passage, traditional medical practitioners, African Independent Churches, and the position of women, are common to all Africans. Hence, this book will benefit any person who would like to learn about the religious experiences, beliefs, and practices of the African people, before, during, and after the coming of Christianity. However, the bulk of its examples will be drawn from the perspectives of the Shona people of Zimbabwe.

Zimbabwe has had its name changed several times. The British South Africa Company that colonized the country in 1890 named it Rhodesia, after the British mogul, Cecil John Rhodes, who financed the Chartered Company. (His remains lie on Matopos Hills, near Bulawayo, Zimbabwe's second-largest city.) During the Federation of Rhodesia and Nyasaland (1953–63) it became Southern Rhodesia, but reverted to Rhodesia after the federation. In 1979, the country's name changed to Zimbabwe-Rhodesia, under the short-lived reign of Bishop Abel Tendekai Muzorewa. It became Zimbabwe in 1980 when its current leader, Mr. Robert Mugabe, became its prime minister, taking over from Ian Douglas Smith.

As has been said already, this book is written from the point of view of the Shona, which is another mammoth task. The Shona comprise the Karanga, Zezuru, Ndau, Manyika, and Korekore ethnic groups. Each ethnic group has hundreds of subgroups, each with its cultural and religious variations. Again, it is impossible for one to write about the Shona as a homogenous group. Consequently, this book makes particular reference to the Karanga of Masvingo, although these are also a diversified group. Despite these isolated differences, the book deals with the general experiences of the Shona people.

Throughout the book, I will use the pronouns he and she interchangeably for convenience's sake, and never as a tool to exclude or downplay the role of a particular gender. The book also refers to the Roman Catholic Church and the Christian churches in Zimbabwe. I am aware of the theological and dogmatic differences between the Roman Catholic Church and other Christian churches. I do hope that the reader will enjoy reading this book. This book is for everyone: students, teachers, professors, Christians, ordinary people, and pastors.

John Chitakure
San Antonio, Texas, February 2017

Acknowledgments

I would like to thank Blessing, my wife, for sacrificing some of her free time in proofreading this book even though its subject matter lies beyond her area of familiarity. I also appreciate all the support she rendered me when I was researching for this book. I also thank Nyasha and Mufaro, my sons, for proofreading the book, and their support when I was doing my research for it. They also drew the maps of Zimbabwe and Africa that I used on pp. viii–ix.

I would like to extend special gratitude to the University of the Incarnate Word interlibrary loan facility, which enabled me to read books that I could never have afforded to buy. Without their hard work, I would not have written this book. By the end of my research, I was convinced that even if I had asked for a book that was published in heaven, they could have brought it to my doorsteps. You are a great team, and I urge all of you to continue doing the excellent work that you have been doing.

I also thank my friends; Professor Kevin Considine for being so supportive, and for endorsing my first book, *The Pursuit of the Sacred*. Sheelagh Stewart deserves special thanks for endorsing my second book, *Shona Women in Zimbabwe—A Purchased People?* There is nothing as sweet as having friends whom one can trust to do the needful. I also thank my Facebook friends for helping me to compose the title for this book.

Finally, I would like to thank my colleagues and my students at the University of the Incarnate Word with whom I shared some of the ideas that became part of this book. These topics were new and somewhat strange to my students, yet they found them fascinating and captivating. When I decided to incorporate African Traditional Religion in my World Religions syllabus, in 2012, it was on an experimental basis. But the interest shown by my students gave me the impetus that I needed to write this book.

Abbreviations

A.K.A	Also known as
AD	Anno Domini (Year of our Lord)
AICs	African Independent Churches
AIDS	Acquired Immune Deficiency Syndrome.
ATR	African Traditional Religion
CE	Common Era
C-Section	Caesarean Section
CZM	Chita Chezvipo Zvemoto Primary School
DNA	Deoxyribonucleic Acid
DVDs	Digital Versatile Discs
Fr.	Father
HIV	Human Immunodeficiency Virus
LMS	London Missionary Society
PHD Ministries	Prophetic Healing Deliverance Ministries
RCC	Roman Catholic Church
Rev	Reverend
S. Rhodesia	Southern Rhodesia
SJ	Society of Jesus
UFIC	United Family International Church
ZAOGA	Zimbabwe Assemblies of God in Africa
ZINATHA	Zimbabwe National Traditional Healers Association

Introduction

Right from the beginning of the universe and humankind, God has never left any people without his saving grace, redemptive revelation, and faithful messengers. God is omnipresent, and God meets people where they are in history, and uses their environment and culture to communicate with them. God belongs to all cultures and speaks all languages, yet God transcends all cultures and languages. Different peoples and religious traditions know and understand God in different ways. Consequently, no one culture or religion can logically claim to have the monopoly of God's revelation and grace to humankind. God is too big to be contained and confined in a single religion and culture at the exclusion of others. Hence, it was erroneous, derogatory, and dangerously misleading for some of the Christian missionaries of the eighteenth and nineteenth centuries to think that they had brought God to Africa, which implied that there was no God in Africa before their arrival. In his introductory remarks to John V. Taylor's book, *The Primal Vision*, M. A. C. Warren had done some serious theological reflection when he profoundly wrote: "Our first task in approaching another people, another culture, another religion, is to take off our shoes, for the place is holy. Else we find ourselves treading on peoples' dreams. More serious still we may forget that God was there before our arrival."[1]

Of course, some of the early Christian missionaries to Africa carelessly trod on people's dreams, violated everything that was considered sacrosanct by the Africans, and seemed to be oblivious of God's presence in Africa before their arrival. They ignored the signs of the presence of God—nature, love, generosity, hospitality, happiness, and the respect that African people had for their own people and the resident aliens. Many of the early missionaries were blinded by the superiority complex of the old-fashioned Roman view of culture that made them think that culture was a commodity, which was owned both individually and collectively. "Thus the entire human race could be divided into two camps: the civilized and the barbarian, the cultured and the

---

1. Taylor, *The Primal Vision*, 10. The quotation comes from M. A. C. Warren's introduction of the book.

uncultured."[2] That mentality deemed a person to be cultured or uncultured depending on the racial group to which he belonged. Since Christianity was considered the religion of the *civilized* and *cultured* people of the world, it was assumed to be superior to all other religions and cultures. The early missionaries' cultural superiority hindered some of them from seeing the footprints of God in Africa, and acknowledging God's presence among Africans, when they arrived and settled among them. Their cultural arrogance robbed them of the humility that is a prerequisite to hearing the whispering and ubiquitous voice of God in any given place. Most of them could not resist the proclivity to condemn most African religious, cultural, political, and social practices that were different from their own.

Armed with the gospel of Jesus Christ and their European cultural superiority mentality, Christian missionaries arrived in Zimbabwe in the nineteenth century, after a disastrous false start in the seventeenth century, when Fr. Gonzalo da Silveira's efforts to single-handedly proselytize the Mutapa State ended up in his untimely martyrdom. In the nineteenth century, despite the warm welcome that the missionaries received from King Mzilikazi, and later, his son, King Lobengula of Zimbabwe, the London Missionary Society and the Jesuits failed to win a single soul for Christ in Matabeleland for over thirty years. When they were finally allowed to fish for converts in Mashonaland, Masvingo, and Manicaland, before and after the unceremonious demise of King Lobengula, they managed to catch many fish for the Lord, but many of the new converts remained faithful to their traditional religion. Yes, the indigenous people of Zimbabwe had a religion that had been handed down from their foremothers and forefathers, which had been providing satisfactory answers to their existential questions since time immemorial. They too had a God, philosophy, rituals, medicines, and theology before the arrival of Christian missionaries. They had beliefs about the life after life. The Shona belief system, like that of most African peoples, was built on three pillars, namely; prosperity, good health, and longevity. Their religious perspective had no hell and heaven, and they had always managed without them. The members of the community who transgressed the traditional religious and moral standards were punished by their visible and invisible elders and God, here on earth, and if they sincerely repented and paid reparations to the victims of their misdeeds for the harm done they would be forgiven.

In the Shona philosophy, prosperity encompasses several aspects. First, the Shona are concerned with the attainment of material wealth here on earth. In the past, their wealth was measured by the number of cows, goats,

---

2. Shorter, *Towards a Theology of Inculturation*, 18.

sheep, and other livestock that they possessed. They prayed to God through their ancestors so that their livestock could be increased and protected from pestilence. They propitiated God and ancestors to have their land fertilized and their crops protected from diseases. The prosperity that they placated God and ancestors to attain was to be realized here on earth, not anywhere else. If God were to bless the Shona people, it was to be right here and now.

Second, prosperity also encompassed their deep spirituality. Blessed was the person who observed the traditional moral standards that had come down from God through the ancestors, and were enforced by the elders. A morally upright person would be rewarded by material wealth, good health, and a very long life. The third aspect of the pillar was moral prosperity, which was achieved by walking the path of righteousness, respect, humility, love, peacefulness, generosity, and kindness (*unhu*). Moral prosperity was summarized by the Golden Rule of reciprocity—do to others what you would want them to do to you, and do not do to them what you would not want them to do to you. A person who has material wealth, lives per the traditional moral standards that were given by God through the ancestors, and upholds the Golden Rule of reciprocity, is a righteous person—a person with *unhu*. A person with *unhu* stays away from incest, ill-treating his parents, marrying without paying bridewealth, killing people, abandoning his ancestral home, and treating his workers unjustly.[3]

The second pillar of the African Traditional Religion is the attainment of sound health of the mind, body, and spirit. Sound health gives quality to life. One can only enjoy the material wealth acquired, if one's health permits it. The Shona realize that good health has its enemies, particularly, the witches and evil spirits. The African's life can be compared to a marathon—fleeing the relentless attacks by the nefarious spirits and their malevolent agents, the witches, while soliciting the succor and the wise counsel of the benevolent spirits such as God, ancestors, alien spirits, and their ambassadors, namely; the traditional medical practitioners.

The Shona firmly believe that poverty is one of the enemies of good health. It prevents one from pacifying the good spirits that are responsible for the safeguarding of people, animals, and the environment. If ancestors feel forsaken, they would loosen the bonds of their protection of the living family members, and by so doing, allow misfortunes to happen. An angry God will not provide the rain that enables the land to be fecund, and may punish the people and animals with pestilence. Poverty prevents one from practicing magnanimity as per the dictates of the principles of *unhu*. In fact, impecuniosity may compel one to steal for survival. The

---

3. Gelfand, "UNHU—The Personality of the Shona."

same poverty may prevent one from paying bridewealth to the relatives of his wife, and homage to the ancestors, which may infuriate the relatives of his wife, ancestors, and God.

Africans, like most people of this universe, supplicate the good spirits for longevity. The Shona concept of longevity can be understood in three related ways. First, it refers to a long life of an individual as a sign of having been blessed by God. This long life enables one to acquire more wisdom, wealth, and to have more offspring. Africans try to nourish their children and protect them from all harm so that they live longer. The ailing members of the society are taken care of to enhance the quality of their lives. Longevity is also understood in terms of getting married and begetting children. A person who is married and has children, even if he dies at the age of twenty, is considered to have lived a long life because his children will perpetuate his name and perform the rites of passage that enable his spirit to become an ancestor. Ancestors are believed to be alive, although they live in the spiritual form. The deceased man's daughters will get married and bring more wealth to the family in the form of bridewealth. Some of the bridewealth will be used to acquire wives for the brothers of the married woman. The acquired wives will bear more children for the family, and the families will make up a great clan and nation.

Of heaven and hell, the traditional African does not know, for he is comfortable here on earth. What matters most for him is the acquisition of wealth here on earth, being of sound health, and living a long life. All the rituals to God, ancestors, and alien spirits are intended to persuade them to bestow their favors unto humanity. Witches, evil spirits, and some alien spirits are dreaded because they do have the power to destroy one's wealth, or obstruct a person from acquiring any. They too can engender some serious adversity, or even death to their victims. The Shona God can get aggravated, if his precepts are not meticulously followed, resulting in him withholding the rains, which leads to the starvation of both people and animals. Ancestors too may allow death to happen to one of the family members if they are exasperated. Death and any other misfortune compel the Shona to consult the traditional medical practitioners. These respected members of the African society possessed the knowledge of the life-giving and life-prolonging rituals and medicines. They had one leg in the land of the living and another in the land of the spirits, and they could understand the languages of both worlds.

That is how things were when the Christian missionaries entered the African scene, propelled by and armed with their founder's ambitious commission, to go all over the world to teach, convert, and baptize everyone in his name. This zeal was tinged with the missionaries' penchant to spread

European commerce, civilization, and culture. The gospel message that they brought was sometimes indistinguishable from their own cultures, and was offered as a one-way traffic that was intended to transform and domesticate the receiving culture, without allowing itself to be formulated and interpreted anew by that culture.[4] In Zimbabwe, just like in other parts of Africa, the missionaries condemned the Shona God of Matonjeni, who had always managed to provide rain and food for his people before the arrival of the Christians. They desecrated the sacred places that the people had always held sacrosanct. They berated the ancestors that had always faithfully protected their relatives from evil, rewarded the upright with prosperity, good health, and longevity, and punished the wayward members of the family. They too had always interceded for their relatives before God.

The missionaries denounced the rites of passage that had always been channels through which God and the ancestors lavished their graces upon the Shona people as they transitioned from one stage of life to another. The traditional medical practitioners, who were the custodians of the rituals and medicines that promoted and prolonged life, were reproached and given one of the most belittling, derogatory, and contradictory names—*witch-doctor*. They also discouraged other indigenous Zimbabweans from learning and mastering the art of traditional healing by preaching that it was devilish. They promoted the practice of witchcraft by supporting the establishment of blanket anti-witchcraft laws that cushioned witches at the expense of the victims of their malevolent activities. As if that was not enough, they handicapped the traditional medical practitioners by legislating that anyone who claimed to have knowledge of witchcraft and dared to name a witch would be imprisoned. They destroyed families by requiring converted polygamists to send away all other wives except one.

The spirit of individualism and competition that the missionaries and their kith introduced and lived divided the people. They maintained that the heaven that they preached could be entered by only qualifying individuals, with or without their relatives and friends. The education system that they promoted was so competitive that it created enmity among people who were supposed to be friends and relatives. They supported the absolute private ownership of goods that was unknown to the Shona people. This view does not seek to portray Africans as people who had no sense of private ownership of goods. In fact, there was private ownership of goods in Zimbabwe before the coming of Europeans, but no one was deprived of using those private goods. A villager could own a cow, and all other villagers would recognize it as his private cow. Be that as it may, that did not prevent other

---

4. Shorter, *Towards a Theology of Inculturation*, 14.

villagers from being nourished by its milk and the fruits of its labors. Likewise, houses, though privately owned, were open to everyone who needed a place to sleep. Many Africans could not understand the notion of a heaven where one could go alone, without one's family and friends, and yet be expected to be happy.

But the missionaries were not fools. They hid the gospel inside their European culture. If anyone wanted to eat their food, drink their wine, wear their clothes, attend their schools, and be treated by their hospitals, then one had to accept their message. They made their culture and the gospel inseparable, and made it a point that they preached to those who came to them looking for European cultural things. They won. The missionaries' preaching was so strong that it forced some Africans to hate themselves. Some started hating their skin color, hair texture, medicines, names, food, songs, dance, and traditions. The missionaries rewarded the converts with goodies, education, and medicines, and separated them from non-converts by establishing Christian villages in which only Christians were welcome. They supported the building of jails in which perpetrators of crimes would be incarcerated and separated from their families. By so doing, they completely disregarded the Shona criminal justice system that compelled the offender to pay reparations to the victim and his family. The Shona could have created jails if they thought they were useful, but they realized that the family of a murdered breadwinner would continue to suffer unless the murderer was compelled to pay some sort of compensation to the deceased's family.

In Zimbabwe, the colonial administrators, who the Shona could not distinguish from the missionaries, arrested and executed the leaders of the First Chimurenga Revolution, Mbuya Nehanda and Sekuru Kaguvi, in 1898. Ironically, before they were executed, one of the Jesuit missionaries, Fr. Richatz, attempted to convert them to Christianity so that they could continue to live happily in heaven after being executed. Kaguvi accepted the baptism, and was given one of the most unchristian names in the history of Christendom—Dismas, the repentant thief. Nehanda could not see the logic of trusting people who would take away her earthily life by one hand, then offer it in super abundance in heaven by the other. She is said to have implored them that if they were so caring and loving as to wish her to live eternally, in heaven, she would rather ask for less—life here on earth. They still hanged her.

The above narrative paints a somewhat critical picture of the encounter between the Christian missionaries and the Shona people in Zimbabwe. However, there were Shona people who, after listening to the gospel message, felt that it made some sense to them. It provided the missing links in African Traditional Religion. Some people saw the benefits of accepting such a new religion. They now had two religious worldviews: their own and the Christian one. Of course, such Christians of dual religious allegiance were chastised for committing syncretism, which Robert Schreiter thinks must be understood from two perspectives: one negative and the other positive. But, the early missionaries understood syncretism negatively, as the compromising of the Christian faith through its illicit harmonization with the receiving culture.[5] The missionaries forgot that the Christian message was not pure from cultural imports. Jesus Christ was born a Jew, and followed the Jewish culture. When he started preaching, he spoke the Jewish language, gathered Jewish disciples, and ate Jewish food. When Christianity spread to other countries, particularly Europe, it was also inculturated into the European culture. The missionaries who brought it to Africa had their own cultures, which they used to understand the Christian message. Now, to admonish Africans for trying to harmonize the Christian message with their cultures was hypocritical on the part of the missionaries. Most Africans accepted Christianity, but still secretly held on to their traditional religious practices. That phenomenon created what Robert Schreiter calls dual religiosity, where Christianity operates side by side with another religion, in this case African Traditional Religion.[6]

I believe that most African Christians have a dual religious affiliation. Whenever I introduce myself as a member of two religious traditions—namely, African Traditional Religion and Christianity—most people are confused. Then, I explain to them that as an African, I already belong to a culture that is inseparable from its religious traditions. The way I was born and bred, my name, the food that I eat, the way I greet people and interact with them, the songs that I listen to, the house in which I live, and my philosophy are influenced by my African worldview. No one can run away from his identity, even if he tries. I sometimes partake in traditional rituals whether I like it or not. But, I am a Christian, and a Catholic, to be precise. Catholicism is a worldview that I inherited. I have two names, one English and the other Shona. I pray to God through Jesus. But if Jesus delays in answering my prayers, I do not hesitate to turn to my ancestors. When God is pleased to answer my prayers, I give credit to both ancestors and Jesus Christ.

I wedded in the Catholic Church and raised my children in the Catholic Church, but I also fulfilled my traditional obligations to my in-laws, relatives, and ancestors. When I am sick, I use both traditional and European medicines, and when I recuperate, I give credit to both. When I die, I want both traditional and Christian rituals to be performed for the repose of my soul.

5. Schreiter, *The New Catholicity*, 62.
6. Schreiter, *Constructing Local Theologies*, 148–51.

I prefer that my soul becomes an ancestor first, then eventually retire to the Christian heaven, when it gets tired of protecting its family from evil spirits and people. If I miss the Christian heaven, like some of us will do, I still will become an ancestor—not a bad thing after all. I firmly believe that he who has two perspectives of understanding and interpreting the world is richer than the one who has only one worldview. I think that my two worldviews make me richer than people who have only one religious perspective.

This book is a phenomenological and theoretical exploration of the African Traditional Religion as practiced by the Shona of Zimbabwe. Although it is impossible for any scholar to speak on behalf of Africa as a continent, considering its gigantic size and cultural diversity, there are certain commonalities that can safely be generalized. Throughout the book, I will use the terms Shona and African interchangeably where appropriate, and will specify when writing about the Shona in particular, or any other African ethnic group. Basically, this book, with the exception of chapters 1 and 9, explores African Traditional Religion, and gives a brief exploration of its encounter with Christianity, at the end of each chapter.

Chapter 1 briefly surveys the history of the coming of Christianity to Zimbabwe, and its inevitable encounter with the African Traditional Religion as practiced by the Shona people. Although Christianity came to Zimbabwe in several phases, this chapter considers three phases. First, it focuses on the seventeenth-century, successful yet short-lived evangelization exploits of Father Gonzalo da Silveira, SJ, in the Mutapa State, during the reign of King Nogomo Mapunzagutu. Second, it deals with the long but unfruitful evangelical endeavors of the London Missionary Society and Jesuits in Matabeleland in the second half of the nineteenth century. Finally, the chapter briefly surveys the proselytization of Mashonaland and Matabeleland, starting after the arrival of the British South Africa Company in Zimbabwe in 1890. This chapter also examines the factors that hindered the conversion of both the Shona and the Ndebele in the first two evangelization phases. It also looks into the factors that facilitated the embrace of Christianity by the indigenous people, who initially seemed not so eager to accept it.

Chapter 2 examines the Shona rites of passage before, during, and after the arrival of the Christian missionaries in Zimbabwe. The chapter focuses on rituals that are performed by the Shona at birth, puberty, marriage, and death. These rituals are then compared with the Christian rituals that were introduced by the missionaries and were intended to replace the indigenous rituals. The chapter evaluates the setbacks that the Christian churches in Zimbabwe continue to encounter in their attempt to eradicate some of the Shona rites of passage.

When the London Missionary Society and Jesuit (Roman Catholic) missionaries arrived in Matabeleland in the second half of the nineteenth century, they found the Shona people worshiping the God of Matonjeni, whose only shrines were in the caves on the Matopos Hills. Chapter 3 investigates the origins and nature of that monotheistic Deity, his responsibilities and that of his priests and deacons, and the way the missionaries desecrated his sacred places, belittled his role, and dispersed his priests. The chapter strongly argues that despite the desecration of Mwari's shrines by the missionaries and the early Europeans in Zimbabwe, Mwari continues to live in the hearts of all Shona Christians and in their Christian churches.

The Shona people had no concept of the Christian heaven and hell, but they had a concept of the life after death. They still believe that when a married person who would have begotten children dies, his living family members have the power to bring him back into the family as an ancestor. Hence, he continues to live, but as a spiritual member of his family. Chapter 4 explores the centrality of ancestors in African Traditional Religion. It focuses on the qualifications of becoming an ancestor, responsibilities, and relationship with the living members of their families. The chapter ends by probing into the survival of the ancestral veneration rituals despite the unabated condemnation that it persistently receives at the hands Christian evangelists.

Injustice, abuse, and ill-treatment of the weaker members of the society by the powerful members, murders, and other criminal offences happen in every society, and each society has devised ways of redressing the losses encountered by the victims, and disciplining the perpetrators. The Shona people had no jails, police officers, and investigators. However, no ill-treatment, abuse, and murder of the weak would go unpunished. It was the duty of the spirit of the ill-treated or murdered person to apprehend the wrongdoers and bring them to book. Chapter 5 navigates the nature, types, effects, and appeasement of the avenging spirit (*ngozi*). Finally, the chapter explores the challenges that African Christians encounter in upholding the beliefs in avenging spirits and the Christian heaven. To argue that one can be an avenging spirit, and be in heaven at the same time, seems to be contradictory to an outsider, but not to a Shona Christian.

Every religious tradition attempts to answer the following existential questions: Why is there suffering in the world? Why do some people get sick? Why do some people encounter misfortunes in their lives? Most Africans believe that some of the sickness, misfortunes, and deaths are caused by other human beings, who they call witches. Witches are evil people who possess mysterious and secret powers that they use to harm others. Chapter 6 investigates the belief in witchcraft, its characteristics, and types. It also surveys the arguments for and against its existence. This chapter ends by evaluating the Christian churches' approach to witchcraft beliefs among the Shona.

The Shona have the power to either transform the spirit of the dead relative into an ancestor if he qualifies or banish it to the realm of the nameless spirits, if he does not qualify. Some of the spirits that are disqualified from becoming ancestors because of one reason or another are not doomed forever, for they can become alien spirits (*mashavi*) among strangers. Chapter 7 explores the nature, responsibilities, and appeasement of such spirits. Of course, the *mashavi* veneration did encounter criticism from the Christian missionaries, and is now at the verge of extinction.

Chapter 8 deals with the traditional medical practitioners, who attended to Africans' medical welfare before the advent of the Western medical system. It inspects their calling, training, types, and duties as medical experts. The chapter goes on to examine the demonization of the traditional medical practitioners as a result of the coming of Christianity to Africa. The chapter ends by exploring the resilience of the traditional medical experts despite all the hurdles that have been caused by the conversion of the African people to Christianity.

Chapter 9 briefly surveys the history, typology, causes, and characteristics of the African Independent Churches. These churches were founded by Africans for the purpose of evangelizing Africans contextually. Chapter 9 presents some of these indigenous churches' rituals as indistinguishable to some African Traditional religious practices. It notes how some of these churches are recruiting their members from the mainline churches, such as the Roman Catholic Church. The chapter ends by suggesting pastoral responses of the mainline Christian churches, particularly the Roman Catholic Church.

In every religious tradition, the issue of the treatment of women is contentious. On the one hand, most outsiders argue that some religious traditions do oppress and subjugate their women. On the other hand, adherents of the religion in question believe that there is nothing wrong with their treatment of their women. Chapter 10 navigates the position of women in African Traditional Religion through the lenses of both insiders and outsiders.

Chapter 11 is a brief survey of the Shona people's concept of right or wrong, and good or bad. It looks into Shona ethics concerning greetings, respect, sexuality, generosity, relationships, and the sanctity of human life. Finally, the chapter compares the Shona and Christian ethical codes.

1

Christianity Comes to Zimbabwe

Christianity is one of the world's religious traditions that have always endeavored to spread their influence to all the people of the world. This ambition, which was at times carried out overzealously by some Christian missionaries, is believed to have its foundation in the instruction that came from the founder of Christianity, Jesus Christ, to go all over the world, preach to all the people, and baptize them in his name, and of God, his Father, and of the Holy Spirit. Being faithful to that mission, Paul, the former persecutor of Christians, who had been compelled to convert to Christianity by the Damascus theophany, became one of the earliest missionaries to take Jesus' command seriously by spreading the Christian gospel to some places outside Palestine. In fact, Paul considered himself an apostle to the gentiles, and he made three significant missionary journeys in which he preached, baptized, and instructed the people that he encountered about the Way of Jesus Christ.

Despite the evangelical zeal to spread the gospel to the ends of the world that some Christians unwaveringly accepted right from the beginning of Christianity, the Christian message did not come to Zimbabwe until the sixteenth century, about 1,560 years after the birth of Jesus Christ. When Christianity finally made its way into the land between the Limpopo and Zambezi Rivers, now Zimbabwe, it came in about four phases, of which three will be explored in this chapter. This chapter intends to give a brief history of what transpired in each phase, and the cultural and religious challenges that hampered the evangelization efforts by the missionaries involved.

One of the earliest missionaries to bring the Christian message to Zimbabwe, which at the time was under the reign of the Mutapa Dynasty, was Fr. Gonzalo da Silveira, SJ, a very industrious Jesuit priest from Portugal, whose evangelical successes were short-lived because of his untimely and ill-fated demise. The second attempt to convert Zimbabweans to Christianity was heralded by the arrival of the London Missionary Society and the Jesuit missionaries in the nineteenth century. This missionary effort was directed to the Ndebele people who had just resettled in the present-day Matabeleland, after having run away from the wrath and vindictiveness of King Tshaka Zulu and the Boers in South Africa. This evangelization endeavor was another frustrating, ill-fated, and unfruitful venture. The third evangelization undertaking, which became prolific, but not without its fair share of challenges, was carried out by both Protestant and Catholic missionaries. This endeavor was heralded by the arrival of the British South Africa Company's Pioneer Column in Zimbabwe, in 1890, and the overthrowing and unceremonious death of King Lobengula, following the disastrous Anglo-Ndebele War of 1893–94. King Lobengula's death was a welcome development to some of the missionaries because he was accused of having impeded the conversion of his subjects to Christianity, just like his late father, King Mzilikazi, is believed to have done.

Father Gonzalo da Silveira, SJ (1526–61)

Father Gonzalo da Silveira, a native of Portugal, arrived at the Mutapa Court on December 26, 1560, after having travelled from Goa, India, through the present-day Mozambique, where he had left his two conferees, Father Andre Fernandez and Brother Andre da Costa.[1] His safe journey to the Mutapa Palace and the subsequent warm reception by the Mutapa and his mother, were perhaps made possible and easier by two factors. First, Father Gonzalo da Silveira was not the first Portuguese to reach the Mutapa Court, for other Portuguese travelers and fortune-seekers had been operating in the country, doing business with the Mutapa people for a long time before the priest's arrival. Some of those traders might have shared with the priest the necessary intelligence and survival skills in the Mutapa jungles that were replete with deadly mosquitoes, venomous snakes, and voracious wild animals. The Portuguese traders had already created rapport with the Mutapa aristocracy, which might have paved the way for the warm welcome that the man of the cloth received. Some of the priest's Portuguese predecessors understood and spoke Shona, the indigenous language of the Mutapa Empire. In fact, one of them, Antonio Caiado, had landed himself a lucrative and prestigious post as the Emperor's translator. He already had the confidence of King Negomo Mapunzagutu, and his mother, Achiuyu. Some historians think that Antonio Caiado was so trusted by the king's mother that he was one of the few who were authorized to sit on her exquisite Persia rug.

Second, the priest took advantage of the Shona's peacefulness, gentleness, and interest in relationships, which have remained one of their

---

1. The Mutapa Empire, which existed from the thirteenth century up to the seventeenth century (1250–1629) covered the present-day Zimbabwe and Mozambique, and had its headquarters in Zimbabwe.

principal characteristics to this day.² Father Gonzalo da Silveira traveled all the way from Mozambique to the Mutapa Court without any molestation from the Shona people that he encountered during his perilous sojourn. Of course, the Shona's peacefulness was later detrimental to their freedom, when it was mistaken for cowardice by the colonialists that came to Zimbabwe in 1890.

A. Nicolaides believes that Father Gonzalo da Silveira had a missionary plan for the evangelization of Southern and Central Africa according to which he would convert the most powerful king in Southern Africa, Negomo Mapunzagutu.³ If it is true that Father Gonzalo da Silveira had any master missionary strategy for the conversion of the Mutapa king and his subjects, he indeed should have been a genius proselytizer. During the period in question, kings had great powers and influences upon their subjects. Once a king was converted to a new religion, the people under him were likely or even compelled to follow his example. It seems that Father Gonzalo da Silveira knew his game very well, for he immensely impressed King Mapunzagutu and his mother, Achiuyu.

As per the dictates of Shona hospitality, the king offered the priest several valuable gifts, and to his greatest amazement, the priest refused to accept them. He was different from other Portuguese men who had come before him. Although the refusal to accept the king's gifts could have been interpreted as an insult to the king's magnanimity, it rather intrigued the king than upset him. Furthermore, the king's heart is believed to have been swayed by the priest's message due to the beauty of one of his possessions— the statue of the Virgin Mary, the mother of Jesus, which the priest munificently donated to the king. This final gesture of generosity from the man of the cloth might have convinced the king that Father Gonzalo da Silveira was different from his countrymen, with whom the king had dealt. Of course, King Mapunzagutu was accustomed to receiving gifts from traders, but most of them expected something in return, yet the man of God refused to accept gifts. The king did not realize that the gift that the priest wanted from him was more precious than any other material gift he had given away before, for he wanted the king's conversion to a completely new religion.

The king reciprocated the special gift that he had received from the priest by offering his life to Jesus. After a few days of learning the Catholic Catechism, Mapunzagutu was baptized and christened Dom Sebastiao, and his mother, Achiuyu, became Dona Maria. The excited king offered the

2. Rayner, *The Tribe and Its Successors*, 34.

3. Nicolaides, "Early Portuguese Imperialism: Using the Jesuits in Mutapa Empire of Zimbabwe," 135.

priest more gifts, this time—cattle, but the priest had all the cattle slaughtered and the meat distributed to the poor.[4] The impressed people followed the example of the king and his mother by converting to Christianity in droves, and as many as three hundred people were baptized. The priest's magic had worked, and his labor and proselytizing acumen had been rewarded. His success is likely to have been celebrated by his superiors in India and Portugal. It is not every day that a missionary succeeds in having the highest authority in the land as his first convert. But the tremendous and perhaps unprecedented accomplishment of Father Gonzalo da Silveira was to be short-lived, because on the night of March 15, 1561, he was murdered, and his body was dumped into the Msengezi River.

Several theories have been put forward for the demise of the priest. One of the reasons for the untimely death of Father Gonzalo da Silveira is believed to have been the influence of the king's advisors and traditional healers, under the leadership of the *mbokorume*. These court officials might have felt insecure and vulnerable for several reasons. First and foremost, the king, by virtue of his investiture, was the most eminent sacred practitioner in the Mutapa Empire. Although he had traditional spiritual leaders under him, he was considered the highest religious leader in the land. The king's shameful abandonment of his traditional religion by accepting Christianity was not only a betrayal to his people, but also a pernicious offense to the ancestors of the land on whose throne he sat. His conversion to a foreign religion signaled the beginning of the death of the traditional belief system. It was the court ministers' responsibility to safeguard the traditional religion of the land, since the king was too young, immature, and unwise to understand his sacred role.

Second, most of the court officials knew that they were likely to be relieved of their positions in the palace if the king remained a Christian. It was likely that the immature king would replace them by officials who had converted to Christianity. If the king would decide to do that, those who remained loyal to the traditional religion would be killed or exiled. Third, the king's instant fascination by the priest's statue of the Virgin Mary, and his subsequent conversion, give evidence of his lack of maturity as a religious leader, and insufficient grounding in his own religion. It was then the responsibility of the traditional officials to keep the young king in line with the traditional codes of conduct. If the king had refused to get rid of the priest, the palace officials were likely to eliminate the king, so as to rid themselves of that shameful scandal. In that case, they would then replace him by a conservative king, who would stick to the traditional religion of the state.

---

4. Ibid., 135.

In addition to that, some historians argue that the principal rivalries of Fr. Gonzalo da Silveira's missionary conquest of the Mutapa king were the Muslim traders, under the leadership of Mingane, who had been operating in the Mutapa State long before the arrival of the priest. It seems that the Muslim traders were more concerned with trade than spreading their religion, and that is why their grievances against the priest were more political and economic than religious. The Muslims are said to have brought before the king some false allegations against the priest.

First, they postulated that the conversion of the king and some of his subjects to Christianity would pave way for the coming of more Portuguese traders and settlers. It had happened in other countries, and there was no reason that would prevent it from happening in the Mutapa State. They also accused the priest of being a spy of Portugal. To some extent, this allegation had some substance because nothing could prevent the priest from sharing sensitive information about the Mutapa Palace with the Portuguese politicians, back in Portugal and India.

Second, they alleged that Fr. Gonazalo da Silveira was a magician, whose powerful magical water and salt would sway the people's allegiance towards the Portuguese at the expense of the king. To add gravity to the accusations, the accusers asserted that the switch from the traditional religion to Christianity by both the king and some of his subjects would bring about drought. In a country where there was no food and human-made water reserves, drought was among the most feared natural disasters. Third, his accusers also alleged that Fr. Gonzalo da Silveira was in league with the renegade King Sachiteve Chipute, an allegation, which might have upturned the tables against the priest. Fourth, Muslims also told the king that the priest was a witch, who possessed a human bone and other evil objects that he would eventually use to cast a spell on the king and his people. It was alleged that the spell would eventually cause the king's death. Finally, it was also alleged that the sprinkling of the holy water on the head of the king would usurp his powers, and render him gullible and unwise. These allegations were scary enough to turn the heart of the gullible king against the priest.

The immaturity and inexperience of the king, which was known to the Muslim traders, must also have contributed to the fall of Father Gonzalo da Silveira.[5] It seems that he had decided to convert to the new religion without first seeking counsel from his advisors. The news of his conversion might have reached them as an unprecedented breach of the traditional political code of conduct. It seems that the king was also weak. If Mapunzagutu was a king worth his salts, he could have overruled his officials when they advocated

5. Ibid., 135.

the elimination of the priest. He could have punished all those people who persuaded him to get rid of the priest. Yet, he was so weak and immature that he followed the direction of the wind. The court officials knew that his behavior would mislead the people that he governed. His immaturity was more exhibited by his agreement to have the priest killed. He could have just expelled the priest from the Court, and revoked his baptismal promises. His acceptance of Christianity was one extreme, and he jumped to another extreme of sanctioning or not preventing the impending murder of the man of God. Although the exact part that the king played in the death of the priest is not clear, there is convincing evidence that he knew about the plans to kill him. Had the Francisco Barreto expedition of 1568 that was dispatched from Portugal to revenge the death of the priest succeeded in reaching the Mutapa Palace, Negomo Mapunzagutu would have paid for his immaturity and folly by his own head. He was lucky that the ancestors intervened through the mosquitoes of the Zambezi Valley that decimated the Portuguese army before it arrived at the Mutapa Palace.

The other factor that contributed to the failure of Father Gonzalo da Silveira's evangelization bid of the Mutapa State was his overzealousness that prevented him from giving heed to the warning of his impending death that his countryman Antonio Caiado gave him. Any normal person could have known that the allegations levelled against him were not only heinous, but also treasonous, and therefore punishable by death. The allegation that he was a witch was also a weighty one, and it seems that there was some credible evidence for that. If it is true that he possessed a human bone, then, the people might have been convinced that he was a witch. In the Shona culture, only witches would be daring enough to desecrate human remains by keeping them in their possessions. Human corpses and bones are sacred, and should not be desecrated by extracting them from the graveyard, which is their sacred resting place. Such allegations should have forced the priest to his defense, or to escape before the fateful night. The fact that Father Gonzalo da Silveira continued to baptize people up to the day of his murder seems to suggest that he was careless about his safety and bent on becoming a martyr.[6] Consequently, his death brought about the premature end to his seemingly promising work. All his labors were brought to futility because he was not afraid to die. The belief that the blood of the martyrs is the seed of Christianity might have encouraged the priest to face his untimely death.

Of course, the evangelization of the Mutapa State did not end with the demise of Father Gonzalo da Silveira, for the Dominican and other Jesuit missionaries also entered the Mutapa State to spread Christianity. Although

---

6. Ibid., 136.

the Dominicans are believed to have stayed for centuries in the Mutapa State, it is alleged that their evangelization efforts were impeded by their corrupt activities and the lack of focus. When they were finally driven out of the Empire by the Rozvi King, Changamire Dombolakonachimwango, their effort died without leaving a trace. When the London Missionary Society and Jesuits arrived in Zimbabwe in the nineteenth century, there was no trace of the missionary work of the Dominicans.

The London Missionary Society

The coming of the London Missionary Society (LMS) to Matabeleland was initiated by Robert Moffat, who had founded Kuruman Mission in the Northern Cape in 1821, and had embarked on missionary activities in the present-day Botswana. It was Robert Moffat who met Mzilikazi, the King of the Ndebele, during the Ndebele's sojourn to the North via the Transvaal, and befriended him. He is said to have visited the King Mzilikazi in 1829, 1823, 1835, and 1857. It was on his last visit to King Mzilikazi when he was granted permission to start a mission in Matabeleland.[7] As a result of that permission, Inyati Mission was founded in 1859, and was placed under the pastorship of Robert Moffat's son, John Smith Moffat, who was assisted by William Sykes and Thomas Morgan Thomas.[8] In 1870, the year Lobengula succeeded his late father, Mzilikazi, who had died in 1868, the LMS founded Hope Fountain Mission. The Rev. Thomas Morgan Thomas left the LMS in 1874, and started his own ministry at Shiloh. William Sykes is believed to have died in 1887. It is believed that the LMS failed to convert even a single person to Christianity in Matabeleland until after King Lobengula was overthrown and killed by the British in the Anglo-Ndebele War of 1893–94.

The Jesuit Missionaries

Despite the challenges that the LMS ministers were facing in Matabeleland, the Jesuits in Grahamstown, South Africa, were eager to come to Matabeleland to do missionary work. They left Grahamstown in April 1879 and arrived in Matabeleland in September of the same year.[9] The king was not enthusiastic about granting them permission to do missionary work in his land. It was not until November 12, 1879, when the reluctant king permitted

---

7. Gelfand, ed., *Gubulawayo and Beyond*, 19.
8. Ibid., 19.
9. Creary, *Domesticating a Religious Import*, 24.

the Jesuit missionaries to stay on his land. The Jesuits, who had mocked the LMS pastors as failures, soon realized that their efforts to convert the Ndebele would be doomed as well. Had it not been for the resilience of Fr. Peter Prestage, who stubbornly refused to heed the order from the Zambezi Mission Superior, Fr. Weld, to abort the Matabeleland Mission in 1886, the Jesuit dreams would have died prematurely.[10] Fr. Prestage's tenacious holding to hope bore fruits in 1885, when King Lobengula, through headman Sindiza, allowed the Jesuits to start a mission that paved way for the founding of Empandeni Mission in 1888. Among the earliest Jesuits in Matabeleland were: Charles Croonenberghs (1843–1899); Henry Depelchin (1822–1900); Charles Fuchs (1839–?); Joseph Hedley (1846–1933); Augustus Law (1833–?); Theodore Nigg (1848–1891); Peter Paravicini (1834–?); and many others.[11] Despite the Jesuits' noble intentions of winning souls for Jesus Christ, they too failed to convert even a single soul to Christianity until the demise of King Lobengula.

For over three decades, both the LMS and Jesuit missionaries failed to convert the Ndebele, even though they had been allowed to stay in Matabeleland and to build mission schools. This turn of events was not only upsetting to the missionaries, but also a proof of the ineffectiveness of their evangelization methods. Several factors have been attributed to their failure to convince the king and his people about the efficacy of Christianity. The missionaries had access to the king, albeit somewhat limited, and lived among his people, yet they could not convince a single soul to cross over to Christianity.

Failure of the London Missionary Society and Jesuits in Matabeleland

One of the reasons that might have hampered the missionary work of the LMS and the Jesuits is believed to be the competition for souls between the two groups. Michael Gelfand notes that there was a healthy competition between the LMS and the Jesuits, which forced the missionaries to double their efforts in their attempts to entice the king and his people.[12] However, sometimes competitions are nasty because of the emotions that they evoke. Although the king was used to European competition in trying to win his favors, the usual competitors were traders, hunters, and fortune-seekers,

---

10. Gelfand, ed., *Gubulawayo and Beyond*, 427.

11. For a complete list of the early Jesuit in Matabeleland, see Gelfand, ed., *Gubulawayo and Beyond*, 26–28.

12. Ibid., 20.

and not missionaries. Missionaries were supposed to be different. They came preaching the gospel of Jesus Christ, the Son of God, who both groups claimed to have killed. Both claimed to be Christians who wanted to convert the Ndebele people to their Christian God. They preached the unity of the believers, and the oneness of the Trinitarian God. Yet the Protestant and Catholic missionaries claimed to be different, and at times, even spoke ill of each other. This happened at a time when Catholics and Protestants savagely criticized each other and overzealously competed for souls wherever they met. The missionaries are likely to have tried to outwit each other to win the favors of the king, yet they claimed to preach the same Christ. Such a divided people and religion must have confused the king and his people.

Suppose the king wanted to convert to Christianity, which brand of Christianity was he supposed to accept without rendering the other group jealousy, thereby damaging his relationship with that group? If both the Jesuits and the LMS had managed to convert some Ndebele people to their respective denominations, how would the converted Ndebele relate with each other? Being a religiously homogenous people, the Ndebele must have found the religion of the white man very divisive. Conversion of the Ndebele was likely to turn the LMS and Catholic converts against each other, and inevitably, against non-believers. Any reasonable king would have wanted to know why the two missionary groups did not unite, since both had come from Europe, and their message of the crucified and resurrected Christ was the same. It could be that the missionaries counter-criticized each other, alleging that the other group was not authentic. If they openly criticized each other, which is very likely, that should have confused the king concerning the authenticity of either group. Even if the missionaries had tried to explain Martin Luther's Reformation to the king that would only have confirmed the divisiveness of their religion. The king must have found it easier to remain neutral by sticking to his traditional religion and influencing his subjects to do the same. Although the competition between the LMS and the Jesuits might have acted to the king's advantage, it dealt a terrible blow to both the LMS and the Jesuits in terms of their missionary visions.

Another reason is that the missionaries, particularly the Jesuits, were unreasonably ambitious and overzealous in their missionary work. The Jesuits wanted to set up missions from Tati and Gubulawayo to Lake Bangweulu, and to Mozambique, a mission that Michael Gelfand considers to have been unattainable.[13] The ill-conceived Pandamatenga mission of 1882–84 ended in utter disaster when the missionaries were massacred by mosquitoes, and consequently, the Pandamatenga and Tati missions were officially closed in

13. Ibid., 21.

1885, having produced no converts. These ambitious missionary adventures exposed the Jesuits to many dangers, and eventually discouraged them from expanding their mission to other areas. The rapid and ill-prepared expansion of missions forced them to thin out their resources instead of concentrating on a single area and supporting each other. The death of some of the missionaries, and perhaps members of their families might have evoked the suspicion of the lack of efficacy in the religion they were trying to sell to the indigenous people. Any reasonable indigenous person would doubt the usefulness of a religion whose God allowed his ministers to suffer the way the missionaries did.

Death not only dealt a blow to Jesuits missionaries, but also to the LMS. In 1862, Rev. Thomas Morgan Thomas lost his wife, Anne, and his child to fever, which left the missionary with a broken heart.[14] These deaths are likely to have caused the Ndebele to doubt the usefulness of the missionary's religion. If the Christian God could not save even the missionaries and their families, then what use would Christianity have to the Ndebele people? The Ndebele, like other African peoples, prayed for prosperity, good health, and longevity, and the missionary's religion and God had failed to protect his own from malaria, fever, and death. In the mind of the ordinary African person, that religion would not be any better than the traditional religion of the Ndebele.

An equally important point to consider is that of the attitude of most early missionaries to Africa. Most missionaries suffered from a superiority complex that prevented them from fully connecting with the indigenous people. They claimed that their God was superior to the God of the Africans, and because of that they maintained that they had the right to convert Africans to Christianity. Thomas Morgan Thomas condemned Ukwali (Mwari) the Shona God of Matonjeni as a fake God who was promoted by cheats.[15] As if that was not scornful enough, Thomas condemned Matabeleland as a place that Satan had inhabited for a long time. He wrote: "In a land like this, where Satan has so long reigned supremely, and where the whole country, government, and people, join their forces to carry out the wishes of the usurper, and oppose everything that is humane, rational, and holy, the progress of a work like ours must naturally be slow."[16] Reading this statement, one can be misled into thinking that there was no Satan in Europe during that time. Thomas went on to condemn the Ndebele king as a despot, who promoted

---

14. Thomas, *Eleven Years in Central South Africa*, 321–22.
15. Ibid., 288–291.
16. Ibid., 342.

war, plunder, superstitions, kidnapping, and slaughter of the Shona.[17] He seemed to have been incognizant of the plunder of African resources by the European nations that was happening during that period. Thomas reached the extent of insulting the intelligence of the African people. He wrote, "It is unreasonable to expect in the native converts the same amount of intelligence or consciousness as in the Christians at home. The heathen habits, in which they have been trained, will still influence them and modify their views."[18] He seems to have been oblivious of the fact that his religion was also superstitious. However, Thomas was right in postulating that the African's worldview would continue to influence the Africans' religious behavior forever. But, he never thought that there was something mystical about the African worldview that made it invincible. His mind was bent on thinking that Africans, their God, and beliefs were inferior to his.

In addition to that, the Jesuits were not to be outdone in abusing the traditional religious beliefs of Africans. They too depicted Africans as savage, primitive, inferior, and barbaric.[19] Both the Jesuits and the LMS did not want to acknowledge the fact that when they arrived in Matabeleland, they had found the Ndebele living their lives happily without the blessings of the Christian religion and European culture. It is very disturbing that the missionaries had the audacity to berate the people that they were trying to convert. It was foolhardy for them to then try to convert the same people that they were scorning. They scolded the same people who had received them warmly, and assisted them in every way that was possible to make their stay comfortable. It is true that the missionaries had come to Zimbabwe uninvited, yet they found no problem in demonizing their hosts' culture and religion.

Furthermore, some of the missionaries might have lost their spiritual direction in pursuit of other hobbies, such as hunting, due to necessity, or sheer interest. In Depelchin's January 14, 1880, letter to his superior, Weld, he complained about Law and Croonenberghs' hunting escapades, which were detrimental to their spiritual edification. He wrote, "The priest addicted to hunting neglects his spiritual duties, neglects the study of the language, loses the spirit of piety and all zeal for the conversion of souls."[20] The word *addict* that Depelchin uses shows that the hunting was probably not for necessity, but just for the sake of it. Depelchin was right that the sole goal for the Jesuits' coming to Matabeleland was to preach the good news of Jesus Christ,

---

17. Ibid., 241.
18. Ibid., 342.
19. Gelfand, ed., *Gubulawayo and Beyond*, 24.
20. Ibid., 190.

not hunting. The engagement in hunting could have been a result of their frustration at failing to convert the Africans. In addition to Fr. Croonenberghs' addiction to hunting, he is believed to have become the great medical doctor of the Ndebele people. In Depelchin's March 10, 1880, letter to Weld, he wrote: "Father Croonenberghs is doing well, and has become the great doctor of the country. Everyday there are plenty of people who are here at our door asking for medicine or begging to be cured of their sores. Even the king sends his queens and his children to be treated by him. Of course, this makes our mission very popular and is a good introduction to get into favor with Lobengula and his people."[21] This diversion of calling must have consumed most of the priest's time. Of course, Depelchin was wrong because Croonenberghs' medical expertise did not convince the king and his people that Christianity was superior to their own religious traditions. Of course, it might have persuaded the king to accept and trust the efficacy of the European medicines, and to permit the Jesuits to establish a mission, but not to convert the people to Christianity. So, precious time was spent in pursuing other things instead of preaching the gospel to the people.

The other challenge that the LMS and Jesuits encountered was their complete disregard of the people's culture and religious practices. One of such practices was polygamy, which had been practiced by many African peoples from time immemorial. There were many religious, economic, and practical factors that had made the practice of polygamy inevitable to Africans. For the missionaries, who had been raised to believe that the one-man, one-woman marital union was the perfect marital union that had been instituted by God, the African polygamous marriages were the work of Satan. They alleged that polygamy was not only opposed to the will of the Christian God, but was also riddled with other defects. According to C. J. M. Zvobgo, Father Prestage compiled a list of the alleged defects of polygamy. For him polygamous families were full of dislike, jealousy, and quarrels, and polygamous men were lazy and had little love for their wives and children, who they neglected.[22] The way Father Prestage put forward his arguments was not only biased against Africans, but it also showed his prejudices against African practices. What he failed to acknowledge was that the familial and marital wrongs that he blamed on polygamous unions, could also be found in the West, among monogamous unions. Those Africans who belonged to polygamous unions must have found themselves being unfairly disparaged by the missionaries. Some of the later missionaries encouraged the polygamous men, who converted to Christianity to choose only one wife that they

21. Ibid., 221.
22. Zvobgo, *A History of Christian Missions in Zimbabwe 1890–1939*, 94–95.

wanted to keep, and to send away the rest. In a country where few women owned property, the dismissal of the excess wives is likely to have caused a lot of suffering to those women and their children. In the eyes of Africans, monogamy was a European cultural practice that missionaries imposed as the will of God, disregarding the testimony of the Bible that they carried and preached from, which was full of polygamous marriages. The most extreme of such polygynous marital unions was that of King Solomon, who is reported to have had seven hundred wives and three hundred concubines, yet he was considered a man who walked in the way of God. The missionaries' message about polygamy was not only divisive and destructive to the African families, but also hypocritical.

Moreover, the missionaries also desecrated the sacred places of the Africans. According to Terence Ranger, the Jesuits offered their first Mass in a cave in the sacred hills where Mwari, the God of the Shona, was worshipped, and those were the hills on whose rocks Cecil John Rhodes chose to be buried.[23] Mhoze Chikowero asserts that, "The missionaries generally located their missions on high ground, often targeting places that Africans considered sacred," and by so doing, desecrating and spiritually disarming the African sacred realities.[24] There is nothing that upsets a people's religious sensibilities as much as the willful desecration of its sacred places. Sacred places are the habitats of sacred realities, and to desecrate them is not only disrespectful to the custodians of such places, but a blatant abuse of the concerned sacred beings. The same missionaries would have offered themselves for martyrdom if the local people had attempted to desecrate their altars and chapels, yet they found it beneficial to completely disrespect Africans' holy places. This behavior might have prevented the people from seeing the value of the new religion, whose messengers had no shred of respect, whatsoever for the beliefs of other people. On top of that, missionaries failed to observe the mandatory sacred rest which was promulgated in respect of the ancestors of the land.[25] Because of such a blatant disregard of the religion of the indigenous people by the missionaries, the natural disasters that were faced by the Ndebele were blamed on the missionaries.[26] The ancestors of the land were believed to be angry and were punishing the people and livestock using pests and diseases. There was a genuine fear among the Africans that their conversion to Christianity would make the

---

23. Ranger, *Voices from the Rocks*, 15, 30.

24. Chikowero, *African Music, Power, and Being in Colonial Zimbabwe*, 23–26.

25. Bhebe, *Christianity and Traditional Religion in Western Zimbabwe 1859–1923*, 29.

26. Ibid., 30.

ancestors and God extremely unhappy, and that would have adverse repercussions for the people.

The missionaries had their opportunities to reach out to the Africans, but they lacked tact during such encounters. On July 15, 1860, John Smith Moffat is said to have preached a sermon that was based on Galatians 3:28, in which he stressed the "equality of all men—regardless of age, sex, and position in society—before God."[27] This message is said to have shocked the Ndebele aristocracy. How could the king and members of the ruling class be equal to the ordinary people? This kind of preaching could not have made any sense even if it had been presented to the Queen of England, for the Queen is not equal to ordinary people. Missionaries knew very well that this was one of the gospel ideals that could not be applied to all people, in all places, and at all times. The Ndebele could not stomach such hypocrisy and disrespect to their social order. Of course, the message might have made an impression upon the lower classes of the Ndebele society, particularly the *Amahole*, but the Rev. John Smith Moffat failed to remember where his bread was buttered.[28] That message had treasonous overtones that might have encouraged the lower classes to revolt against the privileged members of the Ndebele society. John Smith Moffat failed to rise up to the challenge by electing to preach from a divisive and treasonous biblical passage. Encounters such as that could have forced the people to refuse to listen to the folly coming from the Bible. Some Ndebele people argued that there was no need to listen to the Bible since their king could also speak.[29]

Furthermore, the king accused the missionaries of practicing witchcraft. It seems that the missionaries underestimated the gravity of such accusations. Most Africans believe that witchcraft is real, and any accused person, if offered an opportunity, is expected to vehemently rebut them. The lack of knowledge of the African's worldview might have led the missionaries to laugh off the accusations. A witch is an evil person who employs mysterious, secret, and harmful powers to harm others. Historians are not certain as to what the missionaries might have done or said to earn that notorious reputation. It might have been deduced from some

---

27. Ibid., 30.

28. The Ndebele society was stratified into three social classes. At the top were the *Abezanzi*, which comprised the original Ndebele people who had migrated from South Africa. The following class was the *Abenhla*, which consisted of the people who had joined the Ndebele on their way to Zimbabwe. At the bottom of the social pyramid were the *Amahole*, which referred to the people who had been incorporated into the Ndebele society after the Ndebele settlement in Zimbabwe.

29. Bhebe, *Christianity and Traditional Religion in Western Zimbabwe 1859–1923*, 38.

of the things that they had said or preached. The missionaries might have told the people that Jesus Christ, though he was innocent, had been murdered by their own ancestors. That confession of guilt might have been construed as evidence of the hard-heartedness of Westerners, which is caused by the possession of witchcraft.

In addition to that, the missionaries might have preached that the sacred bread that they ate and the wine that they drank were the flesh and blood of Jesus Christ, respectively. That claim alone might have convinced the king and his people that the missionaries were indeed witches. For them, only witches were capable of eating human flesh. This suspicion might have been intensified by the missionaries' encouragement of their audience to eat the flesh and drink the blood of Jesus Christ. In addition to that, their desecration of holy places might have been interpreted as acts of witchcraft. Whatever might have influenced the king to accuse the missionaries as witches, the ordinary people might have feared to associate themselves with the witches. During that time, those accused of witchcraft were severely punished. The missionaries were lucky to escape the accusations unscathed.

By virtue of being the king of the Ndebele, King Lobengula had the responsibility to safeguard the traditional moral standards and beliefs of his people. It was his religious duty to prevent his people from converting to a foreign religion. Like any other religious leader, he was convinced that there was nothing wrong with the African traditional practices and beliefs. His conversion could have been interpreted as betrayal to both the people and the ancestors. The missionaries were too naïve to expect the king to allow them to convert his subjects to their religion without putting up a fight. The king kept his distance from the missionaries for the sake of his traditional religious heritage. The missionaries misinterpreted that aloofness as despotism and barbarism. They thought that their religion and culture were superior to that of the Africans, and that the king was doing his people injustice by influencing them to reject Christianity. They never realized how Christianity had proved to be just like the indigenous religion, for it had failed to save the missionaries from diseases and death.

The missionaries refused to engage in trade with the king and his people because that would have been taken as an attempt to bribe the Ndebele into accepting Christianity.[30] The missionaries were professional in unwaveringly pursuing their mission—preaching the word of God. Although this refrain from trading with Africans was well-intended, the Ndebele must have interpreted it as a sign of selfishness and individualism. The missionaries had access to certain commodities that Africans needed but had no

30. Ibid., 35.

access to. They had guns and clothes, which were scarce at that period, that the Africans wanted. Their refusal to engage in trade with the indigenous people might have been a way of keeping the guns from the hands of the Africans. If the Africans were to acquire Western clothes, it would have made them look like Europeans. The missionaries wanted to maintain the distinction between Westerners and Africans. Although it was professional for them to stick to their core business of evangelizing the people, they violated that same principle when it came to hunting. It seems that they were ready to violate their core mission only when it was beneficial to them.

The other point that made it hard for the Africans to attend the mission schools that had been established was the demand for total commitment from the students. Their type of education demanded an unwavering, and almost everlasting commitment from those seeking education. The Africans were not used to that type of education. The type of education that they had been pursuing all along did not demand such a perpetual commitment from them. They could not commit most of their time to European education because they had other business to fulfill. The young men needed to herd cattle and goats and, whenever necessary, fight in the king's army. Young girls had to work in the fields and gather fruits and other edibles. They also had to assist their mothers to take care of their siblings and cook for their families. For the missionaries to expect such people to spend about eight hours every day, and five days per week, doing nothing except sitting and listening to the missionary's stories, was to expect too much from what the people were willing to give. The Ndebele had survived without knowing how to read, and they felt that there was no need to learn to do it at that time.

The other factor that led to the failure of the early missionaries in Matabeleland was the difference in time reckoning between the indigenous people and the missionaries. The missionaries used the *chronos* (watch/graduated) time, and the indigenous people used the *kairos* (seasonal/task-oriented) time.[31] While the *chronos* time was measured by the watch, the *kairos* time was measured by the task the person wanted to accomplish. The *kairos* time was flexible, yet the *chronos* time was too rigid. Students had to be at the mission school at some specified time every weekday, and probably on Sunday as well. After school, they would be released at some other specified time every school day. There were specific times for break, church service, and lunch. The *chronos* time reckoning was a challenge to a people

---

31. The Ancient Greeks are believed to have had two concepts of time measurement, namely, *chronos* (graduated) and *kairos* (seasonal) time. Most indigenous peoples of the world used the *kairos* time that was determined by the tasks that they wanted to perform. The introduction of the *chronos* time was a big challenge to most of them, and some still struggle up to now.

that was used to the flexible *kairos* time measurement. Before the introduction of the *chronos* time, Africans would wake up early in the morning, at no specified time, to do their chores. They would eat their breakfast whenever they felt they needed to. They would do their work, and rest when they were exhausted. If on some day, they did not feel like working, they would not go to their fields. They were not slaves of their time, for they controlled it. The *chronos* time enslaved them, and some of them could not keep it. Some of them might have missed school or arrived late for classes because they would be doing some domestic chores at their homes using the *kairos* time. Their parents only released them to go to school after they had completed the tasks that they would have been asked to perform. That diametrically opposed way of reckoning time could have encouraged students to stay away from mission schools.

It is said that both the LMS and Jesuit missionaries failed to convert even a single covert until the arrival of the Chartered Company in Zimbabwe, in 1890. The missionaries were quick to blame King Lobengula for their failure, and forgot to examine themselves to discover the things that they had failed to do or had done wrongly. It was naïve for the missionaries to think that King Lobengula would allow them to convert his people without much persuasion. He was the highest religious leader of his people, and he could not just give away his people's souls to the missionaries without a fight. In fact, the missionaries' religion had proved to be as defective, in almost the same manner as the Ndebele people's religion. Missionaries died like any other indigenous persons. In times of drought, their God could not make rain, even for the missionaries' gardens. During outbreaks of animal diseases, the missionaries' God could not spare their livestock. Christians were just as vulnerable as any other inhabitant of Matabeleland. If you want to sell a cellphone to a person who already owns one, you must prove that the cellphone that you would like to sell is more technologically advanced than the one that the prospective buyer already possesses. Failure to convince the prospective buyer will encourage her to think that you are just trying to con her. The early missionaries in Matabeleland failed to convince the king and his people that Christianity was any better than their traditional religion.

The British South Africa Company and the Success of Evangelization

The arrival of the British South Africa Company in Zimbabwe, in 1890, ushered a new and unstoppable wave of Christian evangelization. As soon as the Chartered Company arrived in Zimbabwe, it immediately started parceling out land and gold claims to its members. Some more missionaries had accompanied it to Zimbabwe, and they too benefited from the parceling out of the Shona people's land. The Europeans claimed that all the land in Zimbabwe had been sold to them by King Lobengula, who had signed the Rudd Concession in 1888, in which he was duped into signing away land rights to Cecil John Rhodes' negotiators. Of course, he later realized the scam and his mistake, but it was too late to stop the British from taking over Zimbabwe. The missionaries established several missions in Masvingo, Mashonaland, and Manicaland. Those missions that had been established in Matabeleland remained unfruitful until the Ndebele were vanquished by the Chartered Company, after the Anglo-Ndebele War of 1893–94. It was after then that the missionaries managed to convert the Ndebele, who had been pauperized by the Company after they lost the war, their king killed, and their cattle confiscated.

The Jesuits, just like other missionaries, were successful in evangelizing the Shona. Two Jesuits, Fathers Andrew Hartmann and Peter Prestage accompanied the Pioneer Column in 1890, and helped the Dominican sisters to establish the first Catholic hospital in Harare, which had been renamed Salisbury. They founded Chishawasha Mission in 1892.[32] Father Barthelemy opened Gokomere Mission on the Mzondo Farm in 1893. The Trapist missionaries founded Monte Cassino Mission in 1902. The Dutch Reformed Church, under the leadership of Mr. A. A. Louw, opened Morgenster Mission in 1894, and quickly embarked on the translation of the Bible into the Shona language, and later opened the school of pastors in 1925.[33]

The evangelization of the Shona was not without its challenges. In the beginning, the Shona were reluctant to convert to Christianity, but eventually they accepted the new religion. The people did accept the Christian message reluctantly because they too had their own religious traditions. The missionaries did not understand or speak the Shona language, which compounded their challenges to convert the Shona. Although they were not immediately successful, their hard work and tenacity later paid off, and they managed to convert the Shona to Christianity. They used all sorts of gimmicks to convince and compel the converts to stay in the churches. Some of them established mission farms at which only converts could live. At Kutama Mission, in Chief Zvimba area, they established a Christian village in which only Christian converts could live.

At Chishawasha Mission, the Jesuits also acquired a large farm for resettling their Christian converts. There were benefits of living on such farms

---

32. Daneel, *Old and New in Southern Shona Independent Churches Vol. 1*, 190–91.
33. Ibid., 188–90.

and villages. The believers had access to the mission schools, European medicines, clothes, and security. But apart from those benefits, there were also laid down strict parameters for the residents. For instance, they had to send their children to school, shun some traditional rituals such as *kurova guva*, and had to pray to the Christian God, who the missionaries called Yave.[34] Violators of those rules were expelled from the farms or villages, and would consequently lose their benefits.

There were other prohibitions that the Christian converts had to uphold. African Christians had to discard their evil African names and adopt the Christian ones at baptism. The rituals of ancestor veneration were condemned, and the ancestors themselves were demonized. The Christian converts that were married customarily had to have a church wedding that disallowed polygamy. According to Mhoze Chikowero, participating in indigenous weddings, dancing, and African songs were banned.[35] Some missionaries discouraged their Shona converts from attending traditional beer working parties (*humwe*). The use of traditional herbs to treat diseases was attacked as evil. Their musical instruments were banned in Christian worship because they belonged to the devil.

The African Christians complied with the demands of the new religion, but continued to practice their traditional rituals clandestinely. Most of them were Christians during the day and traditionalists during the night. The missionaries celebrated their successes of turning the Africans against their own religion. But some Africans celebrated their acquisition of two religious worldviews. Most of them continued to call each other by their African names although the missionaries had given them new names. Some of them could not even pronounce their new names accurately. As a result, Mike, Edward, Jacobs, Susan, and Christina became Mhike, Eduweti, Jakuvosi, Sosana, and Kasitina, respectively.

Most of them performed the traditional rituals such as *kurova guva* at their homes when the priests were hundreds of miles away, in the comfort of their mission houses.[36] Most missionaries never knew that the deceased Christians that they would have sent to heaven by burying them in the Christian way, would be summoned back into their families as ancestors, only six months after their burials, or stay in heaven. Of course, some missionaries came to know about the *kurova guva* ceremony, and viciously

---

34. Creary, *Domesticating a Religious Import*, 244.

35. Chikowero, *African Music, Power, and Being in Colonial Zimbabwe*, 58.

36. *Kurova Guva /Kugadzira* is a Shona ritual that should be performed at least six months after burial to bring back the spirit of the qualifying dead into the family as an ancestor. Ancestors' primary responsibility is to protect and guide living members of their families.

condemned it, but there was nothing they could do to stop it because the Shona Christians stubbornly held on to it.

Polygamy also continued despite the condemnation that it received from the missionaries and their catechists. Of course, some polygamists were convinced by the missionaries to send away the rest of their wives, and keeping only one if they wanted to be Christians, as per the canon-law requirement. This demand caused a lot of unnecessary suffering to the women who were sent away and the children that they left behind. Those African polygamists who refused to send away their excess wives could not become practicing Christians. Their refusal to send away their extra wives was motivated by what they felt to be the unreasonableness and illogic of the Christian God, who was so obsessed with the number of wives one had, as if he did not want humanity to multiply. Those Africans who married a second wife after converting to Christianity were immediately expelled from the church.

The payment of bridewealth was also criticized and discouraged by the missionaries. Bridewealth refers to the money, cattle, and other items that are given to the parents or relatives of the bride at marriage, as compensation for her loss, which are used to increase the wealth of the family, and to acquire wives for the brothers of the woman for whom bridewealth is paid. Most missionaries viewed bridewealth as the buying and selling of women. Despite their spirited condemnation of the practice, most, if not all Shona people ignored them. Those families that were Christian upheld and performed both the customary and Christian marriage rituals. Ordinarily, the Christian wedding always came later after most traditional rituals were performed. This dualization of the Shona marriage has remained intact till to this day.

Dual religiosity has remained the hallmark of the African Christianity. This reality has forced some churches such as the Roman Catholic Church to embark on a theological program that their theologians call inculturation. Inculturation means the dialogue between the gospel of Jesus Christ and the African culture for the purpose of purifying culture by discarding practices that are not in line with the principles of the gospel, and purifying those that are negotiable, for the sake of the transformation of the people's faith. To some extent, inculturation has been instrumental in marrying some African cultural practices and the Christian faith. However, some scholars argue that inculturation has failed to achieve much because of its parochial tendencies in which the Vatican dictates what should be done. Consequently, the African Christians continue to have a dual religious allegiance. The next chapters will show how and why African Christians have opted to remain faithful to some of their traditional religious practices.

2

Rites of Passage

Rites of passage are rituals that are performed at certain stages in human physical and mental development to give the participants the courage to shoulder the responsibilities that are associated with the stage reached. Each major transition in human growth is marked by a religious ritual, and its successful accomplishment by the participant and the community to which he belongs, imparts sacred and social responsibilities upon the participant. According to Imasogie, those transitions are public events that should be properly effected before both the visible and invisible communities of which the individual is a member.[1] The invisible community refers to the world of spirits, and the visible community is the living community in which one is a member. Although some of the rituals are held in seclusion, it is strongly believed that the ritual practitioner who presides over their celebrations represents the absent visible community of the initiate. The invisible members of the community are always present. More so, after the initial seclusion of the initiates, there comes a time when all of them are revealed to the whole community. Therefore, the visible and invisible communities are always involved in one way or the other.

The stages of the rites of passage are: birth, puberty, marriage, and death, and each stage has five parts; namely, concealment, crisis, unveiling, celebration, and incorporation. The only qualifications required for one to take part in birth, puberty, and marriage rites of passage are physical and mental maturity of the initiate. Death rituals are performed when it is evident that the sick person is going to die or has died. While the physical aspect of human development can easily be assessed just by looking at the bodily features and signs such as pubic and facial hair, breasts, and menstrual blood of the young person in question, the mental maturity might be difficult to assess. In most African cultures, it is one of the rites of passage's role to test and cultivate the mental maturity and hardness of the initiates. It is assumed that if the initiate can withstand some deliberately induced crises such as pain, loneliness, and harsh weather conditions during the ritual, then, she is mentally ready to move from the current to the next stage.

---

1. Imasogie, *African Traditional Religion*, 52.

Every rite of passage involves the concealment of the initiate. Social anthropologists concur that the concealment of the initiate symbolizes his death to the old life experiences. The natural and deliberate crises faced by the initiates are intended to test their courage, bravery, and readiness to move on to the next stage in their development. The heart-rending and nerve-racking pain that they experience is a reminder that there is a price tag to human maturity and happiness. For example, it should be exciting for the baby to get out of the womb, become an adult, and get married, but there are challenges and responsibilities to be experienced in all these stages of life. It is believed that if an individual can withstand and survive the pain of the transitional period, then, he can survive the challenges that are brought about by the new stage of life he is about to enter. Once the initiate stoically endures the pain that is caused by the crisis period, and survives the possible hazards that are either naturally or deliberately inflicted upon him, he is then unveiled or revealed to the public, amidst jubilation and celebration. Most rituals are accompanied by lots of eating, drinking, singing, and dancing, which make them more attractive and entertaining to the initiates and their communities. The incorporation stage marks the acceptance of the initiated as a qualified member of the aspired stage. The initiate learns to behave and act like other people who belong to the same stage in life. The baby learns to eat, laugh, talk, and interact with both adults and its age mates.

At puberty, the initiate learns the adult responsibilities such as self-care, caring for the family, and fulfilling one's conjugal and social responsibilities. The knowledge that the neophyte acquires at this stage, prepares her for the next stage, which is marriage. At marriage, one can legally indulge in the sacred games of the bedroom, which up to this point, would have been a no go area for her. Usually, this stage heralds the starting of a family and raising of children by the newly married. The stage of death is divided into two primary parts. For the dying, it is a period of unimaginable crises, riddled with fear, uncertainties, bitterness, and the subsequent acceptance of death. At death, the deceased is incorporated back into his living family as an ancestor, after a brief period of concealment and wandering in the realm of the uninitiated dead. The second part of death rituals involves the supporting of the surviving relatives of the dead, so that they may cope with their new world, without their beloved one.

Birth Rites

Now, let us look at the stages in detail. Among the Shona, the rituals of birth begin as soon as the woman is noticeably pregnant. The first one to know of the pregnancy is the pregnant woman herself, who then reveals the good, and perhaps long-awaited, news to her husband. The two usually keep this news to themselves as is normal among the Shona. Very few men and women move around telling relatives and friends that they are expecting a baby. In most cases, relatives may learn of a woman's pregnancy when her belly begins to bulge, or when she begins to wear the customary maternity dresses. Some Shona families may invite their family ritual practitioner to offer sacrifices to the ancestors for the safety of the unborn baby and the expectant mother. Other families just assume that the ancestors, like any other members of the family should find out for themselves that one of their living family member is pregnant, and therefore, in need of special protection from evil spirits that might harm the unborn baby. The period of pregnancy is considered dangerous for both the mother and the baby.[2] The process is more dangerous and mysterious if the pregnancy is of the first child.[3] That is why rituals should be performed to ensure the protection of unborn baby, pregnant woman, and her parents. The pregnant woman may be given herbs and traditional medicines to ward off evil spirits.

Among many other African peoples, sexual activities between the pregnant woman and her husband should stop when the pregnancy is about eight months old.[4] There are several reasons for this sanction. First, the Shona believe that at such an advanced stage of pregnancy, the woman becomes ritually unclean, and too dangerous, just like during her monthly periods, when sexual intimacy is prohibited. Second, it is believed that engaging in sexual activities at this period might disturb the growth of the baby, or may even harm the baby. There is a strong fear that the unborn baby's body might be pricked and deformed by the father's male organ during intimacy with the mother. Third, the abstinence might be out of the respect of the unborn baby, who by now, is considered to be as sacred and pure as the ancestors. In the past, sexual activities between the husband and the breast-feeding wife were not supposed to resume until after the weaning of the child.[5]

Finally, some Shona groups believe that having sex while the woman is breast feeding can cause unplanned pregnancies, which may poison

---

2. Quarcoopome, *West African Traditional Religion*, 136.
3. Rayner, *The Tribe and Its Successors*, 64.
4. Mbiti, *African Religions and Philosophy*, 108.
5. Parrinder, *African Traditional Religion*, 92.

(*kuyamwira*) the child who is being breast-fed. *Kuyamwira* means that the baby being breast-fed would have taken the unborn baby's milk, which may be hazardous to the health of the baby taking the milk. This concept has its origin in the period when modern family planning methods had not been introduced to Zimbabwe. Even now, some African Independent Churches forbid their members to use modern family planning methods. Although some couples resume sexual activities a couple of months after the birth of the child, and may perform a ritual to mark the resumption of these sexual activities, the abstinence from sex during and after pregnancy is no longer strictly observed. It should be noted that modern midwives encourage pregnant women to continue engaging in sexual activities with their husbands, if they desire so, until the birth of their children. They may also resume the activities after the birth of the baby, as soon as they feel comfortable.

Sitting on the doorway by the pregnant woman or any other family member is forbidden because this may delay the baby's exit from her mother's womb. Fire wood on the fireplace must be burnt from a particular end because if it is not the baby's passage out of the womb might start with the legs. The pregnant woman should not walk on planted fields, especially those of groundnuts (*nzungu*), roundnuts (*nyimo*), and beans.[6] The spiritual energy that she possesses at that time might adversely affect the harvest. Of course, she may enter her own groundnuts fields without any adverse results to the crops. She should not look at ugly people and animals because the baby may resemble such people or animals. The Shona call that resemblance, *nhodzera*. As soon as an ugly animal or person is sighted, the pregnant woman should spit on her belly, telling the baby not to resemble such an animal or person. However, the Shona are not worried about the baby resembling any family member, even if he is not good looking, because it is interpreted as evidence that the baby belongs to the woman's formal husband.

The pregnant woman should abstain from eating certain types of food, particularly those foods that have a strong smell, and are believed to attract evil spirits. She must wear loose dresses that conceal her pregnancy from the public, and allow the baby to breathe and play freely in her womb. In fact, the traditional Shona discourage the wearing of tight-fitting dresses by women because of the need for modesty. In the past, the husband of a pregnant woman was not allowed to kill a snake because the baby would be born without eyes.[7] If the pregnancy is of the first child, the woman should be concealed from her parents until after *masungiro* rituals are performed,

6. Bullock, *Mashona Laws and Customs*, 73.
7. Bullock, *The Mashona*, 195.

usually when the woman is about seven or eight months pregnant. The *masungiro* is a ritual that is performed for the first pregnancy to neutralize the dangerous spiritual energy possessed by the pregnant woman, which has the potential to harm her parents. *Masungiro* are also performed to solicit the protection of the woman's maternal ancestors. Before the *masungiro* ritual, the pregnant woman is considered to be extremely dangerous to her parents, that any encounter with either her mother or father may cause serious illness to her or him (*kugura musana*).

When the woman is about eight months pregnant with her first child, she is taken to her family of origin, so that *masungiro* can be performed. In the past, the *masungiro* ritual also had the significance of the acknowledgment of the consummation of the marriage.[8] The father-in-law should protect himself from the dangers that may result from his meeting her pregnant daughter for the first time, by sprinkling medicines on the premises before her arrival.[9] Two live goats of the opposite sex are required for this ritual. If the woman was a virgin at the time of the marriage, the she-goat *(chimanda)* should be one that has not given birth, which the Shona call *sheche*. If the woman was not a virgin at marriage, the she-goat should be one that would have given birth. The he-goat *(chidyamushonga)* is slaughtered and its meat is cooked with medicines. In the past, the parents of the pregnant woman would smear their loins with the undigested food *(mazvizvi)* from the he-goat's belly in the absence of their pregnant daughter, and they would eat the goat's intestines to protect themselves from the dangers that might befall them.[10] For some Shona groups, the he-goat is dedicated to the paternal ancestors, and the she-goat is dedicated to the maternal ancestral spirits. The she-goat is kept alive so that it can produce offspring, one of which would be given to the grandchild for whom the mother-goat was given. There is no *masungiro* performed for a woman marrying for a second time.[11]

Nowadays, some people who live in urban areas may demand the payment of money as *masungiro*, instead of goats. This practice of asking for money is bereft of any symbolical meanings that the traditional *masungiro* had. In cases where money is used, instead of goats, the grandchild would not have an opportunity to get one of the offspring of the goat. After the performance of the ritual, the pregnant woman is supposed to remain at the home of her parents so that her own mother, or any other family relative who is deemed appropriate and knowledgeable, may instruct the expectant

---

8. Bullock, *Mashona Laws and Customs*, 21.
9. Bullock, *The Mashona*, 227.
10. Ibid., 227.
11. Chigwedere, *Lobola—The Pros and Cons*, 18.

mother on how to give birth and taking care of the baby. Some Shona groups perform the ritual that is known as *kuvhura masuvo*, which refers to the widening of the pregnant woman's birth canal using stretching physical exercises and slippery herbs.

Although the pregnant woman should stay with her original family until after the birth of the child, some women may go back to their marital homes after the ritual, but when the time to go to the hospital for labor comes, it is the responsibility of her own people to accompany and support her. There are several reasons for surrendering the responsibility for the pregnant woman to her own people. The Shona know that the first pregnancy is very dangerous to both the mother and the baby, so they want to make sure that if anything happens to the woman her family would not blame her husband's people. They also want to make sure that the husband's ancestral spirits do not interfere with the birth of the baby. If anything happens, then it is the maternal ancestors that would have failed to protect their own grandchild.

The other reason for doing that is to protect the woman from being divorced for real or imagined crimes that she might confess during her labor. Since the first birth is likely to be complicated and difficult, the inexperienced mother might end up confessing to being a witch or an adulteress just because of birth pangs. If that happens among her own people, no one will ever tell the husband's people what the birthing woman would have confessed. Her own family has every interest in safeguarding her secrets. It should be noted that nowadays, most Shona women give birth at the hospital with the assistance of Western medical practitioners. So, any complications are dealt with using modern medical methods such as the C-Section. Once the child is born, the mother and the baby should be escorted to the husband's home without delay to enable the husband's people to perform other necessary rituals for the baby.

For women who give birth at the hospital, the placenta is disposed of in a manner that the hospital deems appropriate. However, for those women who give birth at home, the placenta is buried in the nearest field and covered with ashes. Some Shona groups bury the placenta in cow dung in the kraal, which is an enclosure in which cattle are kept. Other Shona people bury it along the river bank, in almost the same way they bury premature babies that die during childbirth. In the past, the husband was not allowed in the hut in which the childbirth would have taken place until after about five days when the hut had been thoroughly and ritually cleaned.[12]

---

12. Bullock, *Mashona Laws and Customs*, 9.

Although the parents of the newly born may have a name for the baby before its birth, it is not made official until after the falling of the baby's umbilical code. The baby is concealed from the outside world to prevent evil spirits and witches from snatching it. Some Shona people perform more rituals during the early days of the birth of a baby, which are intended to immunize the baby from diseases and other natural dangers. Some ethnic groups delay the performance of more rituals until the umbilical code falls off the baby's navel. A piece of the fallen umbilical code is mixed with a portion of the child' hair and some medicines to produce either a medicinal waist band known as *mutinwi* or a necklace called *zango*. The *mutimwi's* primary purpose is to ward off evil spirits, and protect the owner from witches. Traditionally, the *mutimwi* or *muputi* was supposed to be worn from childbirth to puberty.[13]

The remaining piece of the umbilical code is buried in the nearest field of the family's rural home. Some Shona people bury the umbilical code in the traditional round kitchen. Nowadays, some people bury it in their backyards. This burial of the umbilical code is full of significance. The burial connects the newly born with the ancestors, who are sometimes referred to as *vari muvhu*, meaning those who live beneath the earth. The kitchen is the sacred space for the Shona people in which ancestral rituals are performed. The place where the umbilical code is buried becomes the *axis mundi* (sacred place) for the child from where a radical reorientation of his fortunes or misfortunes can be solicited throughout his life. If things are not working out well for a Shona person, he is likely to be encouraged to visit his rural home, or the place where his umbilical code (*rukuvhute*) is buried. People will encourage the individual in need of a change of fortunes to visit the place where his umbilical cord is buried so that he may reconnect with his ancestors. Usually, the visit alone, without performing any other ritual, was considered good enough to placate the aggrieved ancestors. It is also believed that the buried umbilical code can act as an attraction force to the owner so that wherever he goes, he will always come back to his place of origins.

In the past, other not-so-good religious practices were observed as well. For instance, if twins were born they were killed, their bodies buried in the river or swamp, and the father was supposed to sacrifice a beast to the ancestors through the chief to appease the aggrieved ancestors. The Shona abandoned this practice long before the arrival of the British in Zimbabwe. In addition to that, those children who cut their teeth first on the upper jaw were

---

13. Ibid., 9.

either killed or had them removed by rubbing medicines.[14] This practice too was abandoned long before the colonization of Zimbabwe in 1890.

In the past, the naming of the Shona child was done by bidding, after the falling of the umbilical code. Usually, the child would be named by his parents, but other relatives could also suggest a name for the child. Some would suggest their own names, and were expected to give the child a small gift known as *rupfumbidzo*. Sometimes several relatives would be interested in naming the child, and would make a "bid." As a sign of respect and appreciation, at least one grandchild is named after either grandparent. Usually the names given to children have meanings, which are derived from the experiences of the parents before or at the time of the child's birth. For instance, families that are experiencing many deaths may name their children: Marufu (deaths), Tapera (We are finished), Pasipanodya (The earth has a mouth), and Nyamayevhu or Usavihwevhu (The earth's meat). There are names that signify appreciation, such as Tendai, Tavonga, and Tinotenda. Some names such as Mufaro, Tafara, Farisai, and Rufaro reflect the joy experienced at the time of the birth of the child. There are also names that are influenced by the economic situation the family is experiencing at the time of their child's birth, such as Nhamo, Nhamoinesu, Mudzungairi, Tamburai, Takaiona, and others. Christianity has had its influence on the names being given to Shona children. Some of the earliest Shona Christian names are: Sheunesu (The Lord is with us), Tapiwanashe (We have been given by the Lord), Kudakwashe (The will of the Lord), Teveraiishe (Follow the Lord), Mukudzeiishe (Exalt the Lord), and many others. Nowadays, a new form of Shona names with the suffix or prefix *Ishe*, which means Lord, has taken the people by storm. Isheanotida (The Lord loves us), Ndinatseiishe (Cleanse me oh Lord), Kumbakwashe (House of the Lord), Munotidaishe (You love us oh Lord), Tadiwanashe (We have been loved by the Lord), Tinomudaishe (We love the Lord), and many others.

The traditional immunizations that are known as *kurapira* start with the strengthening of the *nhova* (fontanel) of the child because the Shona believe that the baby's fontanel can be used by evil spirits or witches to make the child sick. Some medicines are rubbed onto the fontanel of the child to strengthen it. Some of the medicines are mixed with some of the child's birth hair, tied into a knot, and then used by the baby as a necklace or waist band. These days, some of the Christian pastors and prophets perform almost the same rituals to strengthen newly born children's *nhova*. The next immunization is against shock (*buka* or *gara*). Some Shona groups use a small creature that resembles a tiny snake called *rujoti*. A live *rujoti* is placed in the dish in which

---

14. Ibid., 11.

the baby is taking a bath, and is allowed to swim around in the bath water. The baby is given some of the water to drink to make her immune to all kinds of shock. Sometimes, the mother throws the baby in the air, and then catches her before she falls to the ground for a couple of times. Usually, this exercise is performed immediately after the baby has taken her bath, and is intended to immunize the baby from acrophobia. Some Shona people place the father's underwear on the child's face, and it is believed to protect him from shock. Soot (*tsito*) from a clay cooking pot *(shambakodzi)* may be smeared on the face of the baby for a short period as a preventive measure of shock. In the event of the baby suffering any kind of shock, the person who would have caused the shock is supposed to chew a millipede, and then spits into the mouth of the shocked baby. It was believed that the shocked baby would immediately regain his consciousness. This treatment is likely to have deterred adults from doing things that would cause shock to a baby.

The baby is immunized against stomach ache (*ruzoka*). Most Shona people use the intestines of a monkey, a piece of which is mixed with water, and then given to the child to drink. Since the monkey's intestines were not readily available, some Shona people kept dried intestines of monkeys wrapped around a stick and stuck inside the roof of the kitchen. Whopping cough *(chipembwe)* is immunized by giving the baby a donkey's milk. The child is also immunized against loss of appetite and body weight. Some Shona groups immunize their children against snake bites. The snake bite immunization is intended to weaken the snake in the presence of the immunized person. Some boys are immunized against growing too much beard when they become adults.

Male children are also immunized against *sexmania*, which refers to insatiable and uncontrollable sexual drives. This immunization is performed during the first week of the birth of the child, before the falling of the umbilical code. The mother of the child directly applies a little breast milk onto the penis of the baby. The milk should not get into the inside of the baby's foreskin because that is believed to cause infertility. This ritual is intended to create out of the boy, a sexually disciplined and moderate man.

The other ritual that is related to the preceding one is the *kuisa mwana pakati* that literally means, putting the child in-between. This takes place on the night when the parents decide to resume the sexual activities that would have been halted a couple of months before the birth of the child. The timing of the rituals varies from couple to couple. For polygamous men, the ritual can be delayed for several months, until the woman is considered strong and ritually clean to resume sexual activities. Some people argue that in the past, the sexual abstinence was for the entire lactation period.

On the night that the couple decides to resume the sexual activities, they should do it when the child is awake. As soon as they finish their sacred business, they should use the cloth that they would have used to wipe their private parts, to rub several body parts of the baby such as ears, nose, forehead, feet, hands, backbone, knees, elbows, and others. After that ritual, the baby is placed in between the parents so that he spends the entire night sleeping between them. This ritual is intended to notify the ancestors through the child that the parents are ready to resume the sacred bedroom activities. The performance of the ritual protects the kid from the shock or loss of weight that may result from seeing the parents during sexual intimacy. The Shona believe that sex has a religious aspect, and because of that ancestors take part in it. During the activity, the man and woman are believed to be the embodiment of their ancestors. The traditional Shona had poems or prayers that the couple recited during sex as an acknowledgement of the participation of the ancestors. These poems were also believed to increase the man's sexual prowess and fecundity, and to encourage the ancestral participation during the act. The Shona call such poems *zvirevereve zvepabonde* and they are based on the totem of the couple involved. The words used in those poems have sexual symbolism.

Some more immunizations are performed as per the child's temperament and character. For instance, the lungs of a sheep may be used to hit the chest of a child who is jumpy and unsettled. This ritual is known as *kurova chifuva chemwana nebapu regwai*, which literally means, hitting the chest of the child with the lungs of a sheep. This ritual is sometimes recommended for adults who seem to be unsettled and jumpy. The phrase is also used to indicate that the person who is being referred to as such needs to calm down, and take things easy.

Now, coming back to the five parts of the rites of passage: at birth, the concealment stage starts during the pregnancy until at least one week after the birth of the child. Although the members of the public can see the pregnancy, they do not see the baby who is inside his mother's womb. The child is concealed from them. During the birthing of the child, the traditional Shona do not allow men, including the father of the child, to be present. The baby is concealed from them until the appropriate time. Both the mother and the baby experience a crisis period. For the baby, the crisis period is that of being forced out of the comfort and warmth of the mother's womb, into the harsh world outside the womb, where the baby is supposed to learn to live independently. As soon as the baby is delivered, she should be protected from harsh weather conditions such as cold, heat, and wind. The child should also learn how to breathe and eat on her own. Most babies are taken by surprise by this transition, and they scream as soon as they are ushered into the outside world. Later, they become accustomed to their new environment, and learn how to survive. I think that some babies wish they had remained in the comfort of their mothers' wombs, where everything was provided through the mother. For the mother, the crisis period starts with the onset of the birth pangs until the placenta is safely delivered. Traditional midwives (*mbuya nyamukuta*) had skills of extracting *(kupindira)* both the baby and the placenta if they could not come out naturally.

The revelation and celebration take place at the same time. First, the child is revealed to the midwife, who immediately shows the baby to the mother. The mother's joy at seeing her baby for the first time surpasses the pangs that she would have endured for several hours. If the father of the baby is in the vicinity, he too might be allowed to see the baby before other people do so. The celebration and revelation continue when relatives come to see the baby for the first time. Usually, they bring gifts for the baby. The incorporation of the child into the family begins as soon as the child is delivered. The child is clothed, bathed, fed, named, and the fallen umbilical code buried. The incorporation continues for the rest of the person's life. At every stage of human development, the process of concealment, crisis, revelation, celebration, and incorporation is repeated.

Puberty Rites

Among most Shona ethnic groups there are no elaborate rituals that are performed when the child reaches puberty. Only the VaRemba or VaMwenye people of Zimbabwe practice the ritual of circumcision for their boys who would have reached puberty. The VaMwenye are scattered all over Zimbabwe, and are believed to be the descendants of the Moor traders who came into the interior of the Mutapa State as traders, and then decided to resettle.[15] Their totem is *zhou*, which can literally be translated as elephant, but their *zhou* is a mouse (*mbeva*), not an elephant. Their sub-totem (*chidawo*) is Musoni. They have two rituals that are almost similar to those practiced by the Muslims, namely; circumcision and the ritual slaughtering of animals. VaMwenye do not consume any meat that is not slaughtered by one of them in their prescribed ritual way. Some of them have acquired new totems and sub-totems. For instance, in Manicaland, their totem is Beta/Ishwa/Hwesa, and elsewhere, their sub-totem has become Mhizha.[16] Aeneas Chigwedere thinks that their greatest ancestor was Seremani.[17] Although Chigwedere

15. Chigwedere, *From Mutapa to Rhodes*, 121.
16. Ibid., 122.
17. Ibid.

does not tell us much about Seremani's origins, the name is not Shona, and might be the *Shonarized* form of Selemani or Sulumani. However, it should be noted that the VaMwenye do practice African Traditional Religion, not Islam, and most of them have never heard of Islam.

Unlike conventional Muslims who circumcise their boys soon after birth, VaMwenye wait to circumcise their boys until they reach puberty. Again, VaMwenye are different from Muslims in that VaMwenye do not circumcise their girls. Even if they originated from somewhere outside of Zimbabwe, like most Shona people did, they are part of the Shona ethnic groups now.

Circumcision is one of the most crucial rituals that the VaRemba perform for their boys at puberty. For several days, the boys who have reached puberty are secluded and concealed in the bush, or on top of a mountain where they are circumcised and instructed in adult responsibilities. They call this ritual *murundu*, which is usually carried out in June or July, during the peak of the Winter season, whenever qualified candidates are available. The cutting of the foreskin itself is the crisis through which the boys should pass. In the past, some boys would die of infection, but such infections have been minimized by the incorporation of modern hygienic methods in the performance of the ritual. After the circumcision, the boys continue to live in seclusion in the camp until they are healed. Before they leave the camp for their homes, they get new names that have cultural significance. All other people are supposed to use the new names of the initiates. If by mistake, somebody calls the initiate by his old name, the initiate and his colleagues should whip the culprit with their ritual whips. Although the whipping is supposed to be ritualistic, some boys overdo it, and that has created tensions or even ignited fights in some communities. In the past, during *murundu*, the boys were supposed to feed on the wild animals that they would hunt. This aspect of the *murundu* has been relaxed by many VaRemba groups due to the scarcity of wild animals. So, the boys should bring to the camp all the food that they would like to eat during the entire period they spend at the camp. If they run short of food, their ritual practitioners may send for more food stuff.

The night the boys return home after the healing, there is great jubilation. It is reported that they arrive at night, at some place where all other elders are already gathered. The parents rejoice to see their children coming back healthy, and having merited to become adults. There is a lot of beer drinking, singing, and dancing. Many more rituals are performed on that returning night. It is believed that a strong bond between the initiates and all other circumcised men of the group, both dead and alive, is established by the shading of blood onto the soil, and the dipping of the circumcised penis into the sacred beer, that is then consumed by the circumcised members of the group. The rituals of circumcision make an individual an insider. It is a sign of one's passage from childhood to adulthood, and in the traditional past, the newly circumcised man would be ready for marriage. He also could shoulder various responsibilities at home and in the community. Nowadays, the newly circumcised young man is still in high school, and marriage is out of the question at this point.

In the past, some other Shona ethnic groups had rituals that are no longer practiced. Some Shona groups would take the boys that would have reached puberty to the river, and would require them to masturbate and ejaculate into the running water as a test for their fertility. It was believed that fertile semen was supposed to sink into the bottom of the flowing water, while infertile semen would float on the surface of the water. Those boys who failed the fertility test would be given some medicines to remedy the situation. On a different occasion, the same boys would be taken up a sausage tree (*mumveva*) and each one of them would bore a hole into the fresh and young sausage and leave it attached to the tree. The boy would imitate to be intimate with the fruit, and leave it still attached to the tree. Before leaving the tree, each participant was supposed to put a unique mark on the fruit that he would have used for easy identification when he comes back later to inspect the growth of the fruit, and eventually to pluck it off. It was believed that as the fruit continued to grow, so would the manhood of the boy who would have penetrated it. When the required size of manhood was reached, the fruit could be detached from the tree, and that would stop the penis from growing any further. One can imagine the fate of those boys who genuinely forgot to detach the fruit from the sausage tree, or of those whose fruits were maliciously and prematurely plucked off.

Although there is no genital mutilation of the girls among Shona ethnical groups, the girls are instructed in the mysteries and intricacies of human sexuality, and learn how to sing, dance, and enlarge their sexual organs.[18] This education is intended to improve the girl's cooking and sexual prowess. In the past, every Shona community had sacred practitioners who were experts in teaching the girls these things. Some Shona groups delegated the paternal aunt *(tete)* to perform those duties, and the instructions were given on an on-going process, starting before the onset of puberty, and ending after marriage. If after marriage, the woman was found wanting with regards to the performance of her duties as a wife and the mother of the family, she was sent back home to receive further instructions from her mother and aunt. That woman is referred to as *mukadzi*

---

18. Parrinder, *African Traditional Religion*, 95.

asina kuraigwa, meaning an undisciplined woman, which is an insult to both the woman and her mother.[19]

Marriage Rites

All over the world, marriage is a crucial institution that is cherished and protected by the laws of each particular country. Each society has established processes of how its people can validly contract marriage. In Africa, marriage is a must for any man or woman who has reached the marriageable age. The marriageable age varies from one country to another. Among the traditional Shona people, there was no consensus as to what that age was, but most Shona groups agreed that the stage of puberty made both boys and girls ready for marriage. However, the Shona expected the wife to be younger than the husband. Failure to get married for any reason other than physical impairment is considered an insult, not only to the individual man or woman, but also to his family, ancestors, and clan. Charles Bullock affirms the importance of marriage in Africa when he writes: "Any mature person who remains unmarried is an object of ridicule and disgrace among the Mashona. He is not doing his primary duty to the nation, which is to marry and beget children."[20] Marriage perpetuates one's family and clan names, hence choosing not to marry is tantamount to choosing death over life, short life over longevity, and finitude over perpetuity.

The first thing that a man who wants to get married should do is to find a woman who loves him and is willing to marry him. Soon after puberty, Shona boys are expected to begin the process of courtship. First of all, the boy identifies the girl that he loves, and then devises ways of how to communicate his feelings to that girl. In the past, there were several ways that could be used to that effect. The young man could directly approach the woman that he was attracted to, and would let her know about his feelings. The boy was supposed to show respect to the woman in question throughout the conversation. Usually, the woman was supposed to reject the initial love proposal, straight away. This initial rejection was not supposed to be taken seriously because it did not mean that the girl did not actually love the young man. All disciplined and cultured young women were supposed to reject the initial love proposal. Any woman who immediately expressed her acceptance of the initial love proposal from any man would be considered a

---

19. Read Chitakure, *The Pursuit of the Sacred*, 112–15, for a synthesized exploration of the birth and puberty rituals among the Shona of Zimbabwe.

20. Bullock, *Mashona Laws and Customs*, 12.

loose woman. A disciplined woman had to reject the initial proposal, even if she loved the man.

There was a way of rejecting a love proposal, yet encouraging the young man to come back again. Some girls would tell their suitors that they were thinking about the proposal, after which they would let the suitor know of their feelings. Once the woman asked for some more time to think about the proposal, most boys would begin to feel optimistic about the future outcome of their proposal. Sometimes, the suitor was eventually accepted after several visits to the young woman. Asking for some time to cogitate about the proposal had some advantages to the woman. First, she would be able to consult with her friends and relatives as to the suitability of the young man. Second, in cases where the woman had not met the man before, she would have some time to do her homework. Finally, even if the woman did not love the man immediately, asking for some time to think about the matter allowed her to change her mind, if she later decided to love the man.

Sometimes the woman never promised the suitor that she would think about the proposal, and would come back to him, even if she loved him at first sight. It was the responsibility of the man to watch the subtle gestures of the proposed woman during the conversation. Signs such as the tone of the voice used by the girl, the way she looked at him, and her facial expression would encourage or discourage the man to come again. It was also the duty of the man to decide if the initial rejection was to be taken as final or not. It was easy to know if the woman did not love the man from the way she said it. Some women would even be contemptuous of the suitor. Other women would tell the suitor that they would not waste their time thinking about the issue since they were convinced about their feelings of dislike towards the man. There was no need for any man to pursue a woman who would have indicated, in no uncertain terms that she did not love him, and would not bother to think about it. However, some young men who lacked tact would pursue the girl, hoping that she would change her mind, which she sometimes did, and most of the time, did not.

Some young men who could write, found letters very convenient in asking out a girl. Once the letter was written, it was delivered to the targeted woman by one of the woman's friends or by the go-between *(gwevedzi)*. The *gwevedzi* was expected to be on the side of the suitor, and would try to convince the woman into accepting the proposal. In some cases, the *gwevedzi* was selected from among the female relatives and friends of the loved woman. These female relatives were considered more influential to the proposed woman, and were likely to produce favorable outcomes in persuading the woman into accepting the proposal. Once the girl received the missive, she was expected to initially reject the proposal. The young man would write several more letters, until the girl accepted the proposal. Some girls would refuse to respond to the letters, and in most cases, this refusal would be interpreted as rejection. Some brave young men would make a personal follow-up to their letters, which at times, fast-tracked the process.

If the woman did not quite know the family of the suitor, the man could lie to the woman about his family's social status. This lying was encouraged, and not considered bad at all. The Shona have a proverb that says, *rume risinganyepi hariwani*, which can be literally translated as, a man who does not lie to the girl he is proposing will not get married. To counteract such lying, many Shona groups encouraged their daughters to marry men whose families were well known to their parents. This arrangement was known as *kuroorerana vematongo*. In fact, most Shona girls were not gullible, for they knew that some of the things their prospective lovers said were to be taken with a pinch of salt. Even if they identified the lie, they would not hold it against the suitor because they knew that misrepresentation of the facts was part of the game. Some men would borrow nice clothes from their friends in order to impress the woman. Again, even if it was discovered that the suitor had borrowed clothing from a friend so as to impress the girl, the act would not prevent the woman from accepting the proposal.

Some shy men who could not stand proposing love to a woman would ask their friends or the women's friends to assist them in notifying the women about their feelings. This service was for free, and worked out for many people who used it. There were always people who were ready to assist shy men to find a woman to marry. Some girls would demand to have a direct discussion with the concerned man before they could make their final decision. At that point, those shy boys were supposed to brave the winds, and meet the girls that they were proposing. Very few girls would accept the proposal because of the word of the *gwevedzi* alone, without personally meeting the suitor. Of course, the *gwevedzi* services were not supposed to be over-used because some dishonest *gwevedzi* could easily sway the proposal to herself or himself.

The Shona culture did not allow girls to propose love to the men to whom they were attracted. It was taboo. Girls had to wait for the man's proposal. However, girls had ways of making known their feelings to the man that they loved. Some girls would frequent the road or path that passed through the home of the man that they loved, with the expectation of being noticed by him. Some girls would befriend the young man's sisters, so that they could say a word or two in her favor to their brother. There were also girls who would share their feelings with their mothers or aunts, who then would begin to tease the young man as their son-in-law (*mukwasha*). Usually the targeted man would get the hint, and would respond in one way or the other. Some men would respond positively by proposing love to such women. Others, would ignore such moves, to the greatest disillusionment of the attracted woman. Although other people could assist either the boy or the girl to fall in love with the person that he or she loved, it was the responsibility of the one being sought after to decide.

All the above methods of finding a marriage partner are still used by the Shona in addition to the modern ways that have been ushered in by the technological advancement in communication systems. Nowadays some people use telephones and the social media to communicate their love feelings to the people to whom they are attracted. Many Shona people still hold on to the rules of proposals, such as discouraging women from making first advances. Although there are many girls who have the audacity to make the first moves, those girls know very well that their actions might backfire, and they may become the laughing stock of the community. *Good girls* wait for the men to make the first advances. The patience is also intended to save the woman's face. Most girls would find it very disheartening and embarrassing to communicate their love feelings to a man, and then get rejected. It is some risky business. Many would rather have the man propose to them first as a sign of his seriousness and commitment. That should be confirmed by the follow-ups that he would make. The man must seem to have earned the woman's love through his tenacity. But the persistence should be subtly and clandestinely encouraged by the woman, otherwise it can be tantamount to harassment. A little bit of wisdom is needed to be able to discern the feelings of the woman who is being pursued before she reveals them.

Once the two fall in love, they are expected to exchange gifts, which the Shona call *nduma*. *Nduma* can be anything, ranging from handkerchiefs to dresses or pairs of trousers. Nowadays, gadgets such as computers, watches, cellphones, radios, and kitchen utensils can be used as love tokens. In addition to that, some Shona people now buy engagement rings for their would-be wives. The exchange of *nduma* signifies the seriousness of one's commitment to the faithful pursuit of the affair until marriage. Hence, in the event of a divorce, the *nduma* is supposed to be returned to the giver. Some men or women fail or refuse to return the *nduma* to its owner after separation, but it is a highly suspicious act. It is believed that such a lover may use that *nduma* to harm the giver through witchcraft. Consequently, most lovers in broken relationships are willing to return the *nduma* to the giver to avoid being labelled as witches. It should be noted that the exchange of the *nduma* is not binding in customary and civil courts of Zimbabwe. It is just a sign of goodwill that can be broken any time if circumstances warrant it.

During the dating period, the man and the woman are expected to abstain from premarital sexual intercourse. Although many young people disregard that prohibition, parents still try to enforce it. The girl is not supposed to sleep over at her boyfriend's home as a precaution to prevent the lovers from engaging in premarital sex. This regulation has become very difficult to enforce because most boys and girls go to colleges where they live alone. After college, they get employed, and live away from their parents. In the traditional past, the regulation was very easy for elders to enforce because people never went away from their homes except when they were visiting relatives. It was every villager's responsibility to make sure that boys and girls did not indulge in premarital sex. The mischievous girls, who disregarded that prohibition were shamed at marriage, if they were found not to be virgins.

The bridegroom had several ways of communicating the absence of virginity to the family of the woman. Some Shona people used a blanket or piece of cloth that was pierced through its center, and handed over to the family of the woman, if the bride was not a virgin. These days, the issue of virginity is no longer pertinent among many Shona groups. Although the virginity of the woman at marriage is no longer a big issue, its absence is resented by the husband, and may lessen the trust he has for his new wife. For some men, the absence of virginity in the woman that they marry may be considered as evidence that she was promiscuous before marriage. The absence of virginity does not cause divorce because men are fully aware that there are many other ways in which a woman can lose her virginity besides sexual activities.

If the woman is a virgin at the time of marriage, her husband would be required to give a heifer (*chimanda*) to his father-in-law.[21] The *chimanda* is offered to thank the wife's family and ancestors for raising a disciplined woman. Usually, the cow is slaughtered during a family celebration. This extra cow is believed to increase the esteem of the bride and her family. It also encourages other girls to try to abstain from premarital intimate activities. In the past, virginity was so important because that was the surest way to know that the woman was not pregnant by another man's child at the time of marriage because there were no pregnancy and DNA tests in the traditional Shona society.

The next step towards marriage involves the bridewealth negotiations between the families of the man and woman. These negotiations are ignited by the man and woman who are in love, as soon as they agree to take their relationship to the stage of marriage. Usually, the woman visits the family of the would-be husband to do what the Shona call, *kuona musha*, which can be translated as, seeing the home. Sometimes the girl is escorted by one of

---

21. Chigwedere, *Lobola—Pros and Cons*, 17.

her paternal aunts or sisters during this visit. The visit is just ceremonial, and may not influence the girl to change her mind. Some Shona groups encourage those intending to get married to visit the paternal aunt to receive instructions on how to go about the marriage negotiations. She may assist them in identifying the go-between, known as *munyayi* or *dombo*. Usually, the *munyayi* should be a respectable friend (*sahwira*) of the father-in-law. Once the *munyayi* is identified, and agrees to perform the intermediary duties, the family members of the man then accompany the *munyayi* to the home of the woman on the date that would have been set by the *munyayi* and the woman's relatives. The would-be husband does not need to be present on the first round of talks. If this marriage is a *kukumbira* type, the woman is still living with her family at this point.[22] If she is already living with her husband, or alone, elsewhere, she has to be present during the first round of bridewealth negotiations. After paying for the permission to enter the homestead of the woman's father, brother or guardian, the man's delegation may be allowed to enter one of the houses allocated to them by the woman's family. Ordinarily, the man's delegation includes his brothers, friends, and paternal aunt, or sister. The man himself is encouraged to be present, but the negotiations may be carried out in his absence. His presence is a big advantage to the negotiators, since it will be his money being used. However, if present, he is supposed to remain passive throughout the negotiations so that his elders may do the negotiations.

After all the miscellaneous payments and *rugaba* have been charged, bargained for, and paid, the family of the woman may allow the groom's delegation to enter the house in which they are sitting, so that they do the introductions. Up to this point, the *munyayi* would be plying the route between the two houses in which the two families are separately housed, and it is through the *munyayi* that the families carry out the bridewealth negotiations. The son-in-law and his delegation greets the relatives of the woman after each one of them has been introduced by the family's spokesperson. There is a lot of clapping of hands (*gusvi*) as a sign of respectful greeting to every person who is being introduced. Some young men would have rehearsed this type of hands clapping, a couple of weeks before the negotiations. The man's delegation should not sit on the chairs even if they are offered because it is considered disrespectful to the woman's family. In the past, the son-in-law was supposed to sit on the floor, behind the slightly opened door, where very few people could see him. Nowadays many families do not oblige the son-in-law to sit behind the door.

---

22. For a detailed description of Shona marriage types, read Chitakure, *Shona Women in Zimbabwe*, chapters 2–3.

Bridewealth Charges

At the onset of the negotiations, the woman being married is asked by the head of her family delegation if she knows and loves the man who wants to marry her, so that they may charge and accept the bridewealth. The obvious answer is affirmative, and once that is confirmed, the bridewealth negotiations may start. The parts and items of bridewealth vary from one place to another. However, the basics are similar among most Shona ethnic groups. The first part of the bridewealth is called *vhuramuromo*, which literally means opening one's mouth to begin the negotiations. This amount is paid before the man's delegation is allowed into the home of their father-in-law (*vatezvara*). As soon as the *vhuramuromo* is paid, the *kupinda mumusha* (entering the home) payment is requested. This amount gives the man's delegation the permission to enter the homestead of the woman's family.

The next charges, which are known as *zvibinge*, are presented to the man's delegation in the form of a list. These charges are penalties for the misdemeanors and violations that both the woman and the man intending to get married might have committed. One of these charges is called *mapfukudza dumbu* that is given to the mother-in-law for her loss of the girlish bodily form after giving birth to the girl who is being married. It is also paid to compensate the mother-in-law for the discomfort that she might have experienced due to the kicking about, that the woman who is being married would have done inside the womb of her mother during her pregnancy. *Kupfukudza* means carelessly kicking about, and *dumbu* is the womb or belly. In the past *mapfukudza dumbu* was only paid for the first-born girl child only, but nowadays it is paid for any girl being married.

The mother-in-law also gets some payment for formalizing her relationship with the son-in-law, who up to this point would not have been permitted to greet her. This payment is called *mari yegusvi*, which refers to the money paid to acquire the permission to greet someone by clapping hands, while kneeling.[23] From this day on, the *gusvi* becomes the customary mode of greeting that the son-in-law uses whenever he greets the mother-in-law. Most Shona groups do not allow the shaking of hands between the *ambuya and mukwasha*. The *gusvi* greeting is also reserved for all the brothers-in-law's wives, who are practically more revered than the mother-in-law. The Karanga refer to them as *ambuya* because any one of their daughters can become the son-in-law's second wife, if need be. Another payment that the mother-in-law gets is called *mushonga* (medicines),

---

23. Gelfand, *Shona Ritual*, 182.

and refers to the bitter herbs that she would have chewed for the woman when she was too young to chew her own medicines.[24]

Included in the *zvibinge* list is *bwanya zhowa*, which literally means, breaking the fence. This payment is a penalty for the moments when the man would have secretly visited the girl through unorthodox homestead entrances. This amount should be paid even if the man never visited the woman at her home in the period before bridewealth negotiations. *Matekenya ndebvu*, (scratching one's beard), which is charged for two issues then follows. First, it compensates *vatezvara* (father-in-law) for the time the woman who is being married played with her father's beard as a baby. Second, it compensates the father-in-law for the time he spent scratching his beard during difficult times when he was thinking about the ways in which to support his family. The *mukwasha* is also charged the beast of *makandihwa nani* (how did you know about my daughter?), which queries the *mukwasha* about how he came to know of the woman he is marrying. Nowadays, most families opt to receive this beast in monetary form.

After all the *zvibinge* have been paid, the woman's family may ask the son-in-law's delegation to bring in the groceries. Usually, the man would have received a list of the needed items a couple of weeks before the marriage negotiations. The items may include, but not limited to the following: bread, soft drinks, beer, sugar, salt, meat, match sticks, rice, tea leaves, powdered milk, and dried fish. These items should be provided in large quantities, and will be used by the family of the woman. In recent years, there have been reports of families that ask for cellphones and other modern technological gadgets. The payment of grocery is a new phenomenon among some Karanga groups of Masvingo. In the past, the Karanga had the *mafundo* (feasting) that was reciprocated by both families. It should be noted that the *zvibinge* and groceries are not considered to be bridewealth proper, and in the event of a divorce, they are not supposed to be refunded. All the above charges may amount to about four thousand United States of America dollars, and that will be just the beginning.

After most of the *zvibinge* have been paid, and the groceries accepted, the payment of the bridewealth proper, begins. *Rugaba* or *rutsambo* is the first of those payments. *Rugaba* refers to the tin that was used as a cup for water and beer drinking. *Rutsambo* refers to a grass bangle used by many traditional Shona women as a wrist adornment. *Rugaba* gives the mukwasha two marital rights. First, it gives the *mukwasha* exclusive sexual access to the woman who he is marrying. Second, its payment allows the *mukwasha* to take charge of the productive capacity of the woman. Usually, *rugaba* is

---

24. Ibid., 182.

charged in cash, and the amount paid depends on the economic status of the husband, and the *quality* of the woman being married. In the past, virgins were considered qualitatively superior to non-virgins, and consequently, fetched more *rugaba*.

Nowadays, the educated women do fetch more *rugaba*, since it is believed that they will enrich the families of their husbands. Although the *rugaba* can be negotiated, some families do not accept bargains in its payment. What is charged is usually non-negotiable. Again, the son-in-law is expected to pay the amount asked in full. However, if the man is unable to pay the full sum of *rugaba*, some families accept its partial payment in anticipation of receiving the arrears soon. This charge is crucial because it gives the husband exclusive sexual access to his wife. Any sexual encounter between the man and woman before a substantial amount of *rugaba* has been paid is considered unlawful. Technically, once the payment has been accepted, the man and woman may consummate their marriage. Of course, the consummation of a Shona marriage is a long process that starts with the initial sexual act, and is sealed by the birth of a sufficient number of children.

Once *rugaba* is paid, either in full or in part, the next payment is *danga*, which refers to the head of cattle. This payment is for the husband's entitlement to the children. In the past, the payment was supposed to be in cows only. Nowadays, *danga* is charged in cows, but some of the cows are payable in monetary form. The cows charged are about ten in number. The required live cows' payment must be pegged at the market price of a cow at that time, in the area where the woman's family lives. In the event of the price of a cow increasing, the *vatezvara* may also adjust the amount for each outstanding cow to suit the market price. The men whose families own cattle may opt to pay for *danga* using live cattle. If the son-in-law is required to give his father-in-law four live beasts, whose price is pegged at the market price of a beast in that area, he may pay a nominal fee, usually below the market value of a cow, for the outstanding cows.

There are other payments connected to the *danga*, one of which is *munongedzo* (pointing stick or finger) or *maziso* (eyes), which is charged for the finger or stick that is used to point at the cows, and the eyes that the father-in-law uses to see the cows for the first time, when they are being presented to him. In some places, *munongedzo* and *maziso* may be charged separately. *Makwiradanga* is the amount that is charged for the *tezvara's* risk in climbing up the kraal (cattle pen) to see the cows. *Shamhu*, which means stick, is paid for the whip that *vatezvara* would use to drive the cows back to his village. In the past, the head of cattle was supposed to be preceded by a Billy-goat (*nhungamiradanga*).²⁵ This goat would be slaughtered, and its meat consumed by the father-in-law and the people who would assist him to drive the cattle back to his village. The *mukwasha* is not expected to pay all the *danga* on the same day, even if he can afford to do so. He may pay a few cows, and then promise to pay the remainder, later.

Danga is paid for the entitlement to the children that will be born in that marriage union, and the birth of children will consummate the marriage. Many parents are reluctant to accept the full *danga* before their daughter fulfills the responsibility of fecundity because if a woman for whom *danga* was paid fails to give birth to children, then her parents have the obligation to offer the *mukwasha* another wife, particularly the woman's young sister or her brother's daughter, if requested by the *mukwasha*. If they do not want to make that offer, then part of the bridewealth has to be returned to the *mukwasha* to enable him to use it for another wife who would bear children for him. Nowadays, the refunding of bridewealth is no longer popular because most men can afford to pay bridewealth for another wife without asking for a refund from their former fathers-in-law.

In addition to the cattle that the *vatezvara* (father-in-law) charges, there is only one cow that should be given to the mother-in-law. This sacred cow is popularly known as *mombe youmai* (beast of motherhood). This cow should be a live heifer, and is dedicated to the maternal ancestors. It belongs to the wife's mother, and in the event of a divorce between the mother-in-law and father-in-law, the mother-in-law retains her cow and its offspring. If the mother-in-law dies, the ownership of the cows passes to her own relatives. After the cow produces about three cows, the mother-in-law should invite the *mukwasha* and his family for a ritual in which one of the offspring of the beast of motherhood is sacrificed to appease the maternal ancestors. This ritual should be carried out as long as there is a living offspring of the son-in-law and the woman for which it was paid.²⁶ These days, some mothers-in-law ignore this ritual because of greed or ignorance. The beast of motherhood is a gift to the maternal ancestors to solicit their blessings and protection of the granddaughter and her children. So, occasionally, one of the offspring of the cow should be offered to the ancestors, and failure to do that renders the payment of the beast futile. Sometimes, the *mukwasha* may send the *munyayi* to remind the mother-in-law of the need to perform the ritual. The beast of motherhood is not necessarily paid on the day of bridewealth negotiations. Usually, it is paid later after the married woman

---

25. Ibid., 172.
26. Chigwedere, *Lobola—Pros and Cons*, 20.

would have given birth to a child. At that time, the father-in-law would have received several of the *danga* cows.

The last part of bridewealth is the *majasi* or *mabhachi*, which refer to coats and suits that are bought for *vatezvara* and the mother-in-law. The *mukwasha* is furnished with the clothes sizes of the in-laws. The *majasi* items include: a suit for the father-in-law, which includes, a jacket, shirt, pair of trousers, tie, shoes, socks, and an overcoat, and another suit for the mother-in-law, which includes, jacket, skirt, head veil, shoes, blanket, a rug, jug, and an overcoat. These items are delivered later during the course of the marriage. The primary purpose of *majasi* is to make the parents of the wife presentable. The parents are supposed to receive these items from all their married daughters. In the past, these items were not refundable if there was a divorce between their daughter and her husband because they are not considered to be part of the proper bridewealth.

It is very interesting to note that bridewealth is not buying and selling of women. All the charges refer to the services that the woman will provide, but the woman herself remains a free person. There is no price tag on her soul, and she remains a member of her family of origin. She keeps her own totem and sub-totem. In the event of her death, her own people are responsible for performing her burial rites. If her people refuse to perform those burial rites, then the spirit of the dead woman would come back as an avenging spirit to seek justice from her husband's family. The fear of such a spirit encourages most Shona men to pay bridewealth for their wives. In fact, no Shona marriage is considered valid, customarily, unless bridewealth is paid. No Shona woman is comfortable in a marriage, unless bridewealth is paid. Church weddings and civil marriages that are not sanctioned by the woman's family are not considered valid by the woman's relatives, unless part of the bridewealth is paid. When the woman dies, it is the duty of her sons to provide funds for the cleansing ritual that transforms her spirit into an ancestor, but her own relatives preside over the performance of the ritual.

After the successful bridewealth negotiation and the payment of some of it, the woman may then be escorted to her husband's home. In the past, a big celebration called *mutimba* would be performed at both the wife's and husband's homes. At that ritual, people sang, ate, and danced. Gifts were also offered to the newly-weds. The woman's team would be singing songs that praised the woman, and denigrated the husband and his family. The husband's team would be doing the same to the wife's team. For instance, one of the songs that could be sung by the wife's delegation is:

"Margie here.

Margie mwanangu.

Mwana wechinoto.

Wakanga washaya.

Kunyengwa kwaChitakure.

Kusina neimba.

Tondorara pai.

Tondorara mutsapi.

Mune magadzinda."

The words of the above song can be translated as, "Margie, what were you missing, to be married to the Chitakures, where there is not even a house. Where shall we sleep? We will sleep in a granary that is full of bedbugs."

The husband's team could respond by singing a song such as:

"Ndineurombo nehama yedu.

Yakarooara chimukakwindi.

Chinobika sadza mbodza.

Nekanyama kane honye"

The above song can be translated as, "I feel pity for our kin, who married a lazy woman. A woman who serves half-cooked food with rotten meat that has fagots."

This teasing game would go on as long as the celebration lasted. These insults were not supposed to be taken seriously because they were not based on facts, and were intended to be jokes. They were didactic in nature, instructing the couple to avoid being mean people in their new home. During the celebration, and a few days after it, the daughter-in-law (*muroora*) was supposed to cover her head and face with a cloth, and would only unveil it for the person who would have offered her a gift. The *muroora* is also supposed to give warm, face washing water to all the relatives of the husband. Early in the morning, she is accompanied by her own sisters or friends, and take with them warm water, soap, towel, dish, body lotion, and visit the homes of the husband's relatives to offer them water to wash their faces. After the ritual, the *muroora* may be offered gifts.

The Shona believe that every marriage must be fruitful, meaning that children should be born out of it. After having facilitated and negotiated the marriage and bridewealth of the couple, both families look forward to the arrival of children. Parents of both the man and the woman are anxious about any delay in this consummation of a Shona marriage. The man and his people want children to bless the marriage for the perpetuation of the family name, and for carrying out the rituals that prolong the parents' lives as ancestors. Usually the Shona are not quite concerned about the gender of the first grandchild since they expect more children to be born. With the birth of the first born, they celebrate the evidence of the woman's fecundity, and are convinced that male children would follow. If the first child is a boy, the merrier they are because they already have someone to perpetuate the family name and to keep them in remembrance as ancestors. This remembrance prolongs one's period as an ancestor.

The preference of having the boy child early in marriage does not mean that the girl child is not valued, for both girls and boys are important to the Shona people. However, boys and girls have different responsibilities. Since, the roles of the sons are more crucial to the longevity of the family name, and the transformation of the dead parents into ancestors, failure to have male children may bring instability to a Shona marriage. The birth of children consummates the Shona marriage, but the arrival of male children makes the union stead and solid. Girls are crucial because they take care of their parents and siblings. In the past, some of the bridewealth paid for them would be used to pay bridewealth for the wives of their brothers. Their children (*vazukuru*) are sacred practitioners in religious issues concerning their maternal grandparents, uncles, and aunts.

The challenges of barrenness to any married African woman are unimaginable. Without the marriage being sealed by the birth of children, it can be easily dissolved, or the husband may have an easy excuse to take another wife, or to involve himself in extramarital affairs. Charles Bullock succinctly captures the horrors of a barren Shona woman. He writes, "Barrenness is more bitter than death; but the shame of that state is as nought compared to the bleak despair brought by the slow killing of the hope that a child may be given to her."[27] The failure by the woman to bear children does not necessarily lead to divorce. Her parents are not immediately asked to return the bridewealth that they would have received. The barren woman is not considered completely useless because her husband continues to enjoy some of the rights for which he would have paid bridewealth. For instance, he still enjoys conjugal rights. However, in the past, most fathers-in-law felt obligated to make another wife available to the son-in-law, particularly their daughter's young sister, so that she can bear children for her sister. This was more reasonable if the son-in-law would have paid *danga,* which gives him the entitlement to children born out of that marriage. In the cases of women

---

27. Bullock, *The Mashona*, 11.

for whom no *danga* would have been paid, the woman's family might not ask the son-in-law to pay the arrears, if they are not ready to provide him with another fruitful wife.

The offer of another wife prevented the son-in-law from seeking another wife elsewhere. The father-in-law still received bridewealth for their daughter who is offered as a second wife to their son-in-law. In the Shona culture, a married woman's young sisters and nieces (her brothers' daughters) are considered *wives-in-waiting* for the *mukwasha*. In the event of the woman's premature death, any one of her sisters or nieces could easily be offered as a wife to the widower, so that she carries out the marital responsibilities left unfinished by her sister. Hubert Bucher calls a woman given to marriage to replace her deceased sister or to bear children for a barren one, a "substitute" wife, who the wife-givers should offer to the wife-receivers to avoid returning a proportionate part of the bridewealth.[28] Hence, barrenness on the part of the woman is devastating, and heralds an unstable marriage. However, there are many Shona men who continue to love and support their wives, even if they are barren. Many men never try to marry a second wife, and may refuse to take the offered *muramu* (wife's young sister) as either *chimutsamapfihwa* or *chigadzamapfihwa* (replacement wife), although that is considered an insult to the ancestors.

Among the Shona, the infertility of a man is a horrible and devastating thing to happen. All men are believed to be fecund and able to bear children. The Shona call the man who is infertile, *ngomwa*, which sounds derogatory. To refer to a Shona man as *ngomwa* is an insult that might not be forgivable, even if it is a fact. In the past, whenever a newly married couple failed to get a child, the first suspect was the woman. Since there were no foolproof fertility tests carried out, the woman had to bear the wrath of the husband's relatives until her innocence was ascertained. However, if the man was a *ngomwa*, sooner or later his relatives would know about it. If all efforts of enhancing his fertility through herbs failed, the man's family would make secret arrangements with one of his young brothers to have a clandestine sexual affair with his brother's wife for bearing children for him. The children born out of that affair belonged to the formal husband. It should be noted that this affair was not intended to be romantic, but the fulfillment of one's duties.

Most women who found themselves in that situation did not object to that arrangement since it was not considered to be adultery. The woman did not need to have any love feelings for the husband's brother. She only needed to be receptive to and cooperative with her husband and family's

---

28. Bucher, *Spirits and Power*, 62.

arrangements. This secret was not communicated to the woman's family because it would embarrass both their daughter and her husband. If they got to know about it, the arrangement would give them some relief because their daughter would have an opportunity to fulfill her child-bearing responsibility. This arrangement was a way of saving the marriage by assisting the childless couple getting the kids of their own. Nowadays, many men would rather remain childless than accepting a secret sexual affair between one of their brothers and their wives.

Most Westerners who face the challenge of childlessness would think of adopting a child, but adoption is not an option for the Shona people. For them, children should be born to their parents, not adopted. Of course, the Shona people usually take care of their relatives' children because they have a responsibility to do that, but those children remain their parents' children. Most Shona people would rather die childless than officially adopting a child. Even if they were to adopt kids, those kids would be unqualified to carry out the rituals that would prolong the adopting parents' lives as ancestors, because the adopted kids are not their biological children. More so, the adopted children are likely to have different totems and ancestors from those of the adopting parents.

The Shona marriage can be dissolved whenever it becomes necessary to do so. However, before a divorce can take place, all interested parties' concern is to save the marriage. All marital challenges are forgivable although barrenness and repeated unfaithfulness of the woman extremely make the marriage vulnerable. However, in circumstances where reconciliation is not in the best interest of the couple, the husband is supposed to give his wife a token of divorce. In the traditional past, the token could be a chicken or any other small gift. When the economy was monetarized, money (as little as a dollar) could be used as a token of divorce. This token is known as *gupuro*, a noun from the Shona verb *kukupura*, which means to wipe off, as in wiping sweat using one's hand. The *gupuro* is used by the woman as evidence to her own people that she indeed has been divorced. A woman who could not show *gupuro* to her relatives, as evidence of her divorce would not be considered divorced. Most women who were fed up by their marital unions and wanted divorce would demand for *gupuro* from their husbands. Nowadays, *gupuro* can be several hundreds of United States dollars, and might not be offered or asked for, since most women can take care of themselves after divorce.

Gupuro is normally paid by men, not women. In the traditional past, very few women had valid reasons to divorce their husbands, and they were not expected to give the husband the token of divorce. One of the justified reasons for which a woman could divorce her husband was provable impotency of the husband.[29] The Shona call this impotency, *kushaya moto*, which literally means, the lack of fire, from the husband. The husband could also be divorced if he committed incest, or killed a child or relative.[30] The *gupuro* can be revoked if the couple decides to reconcile. In that case, the woman should return the *gupuro* to the husband to signify a fresh start. Traditionally, the wife could be divorced for barrenness, incorrigibility, and refusal to grant conjugal rights to the husband.[31]

The payment of *danga* ensures the husband the entitlement to the children. If there is a divorce, the children should stay with their father. If the couple has children that still rely on the mother for basic sustenance, they are supposed to go with the mother, and are expected to come back to their father later, after a token of gratitude *(uredzwa)* has been paid to the guardian of the ex-wife. The children can visit either parent without much restriction. If any of the female children gets married, the father receives the bridewealth. However, the divorced mother is supposed to be involved in the bridewealth negotiations, so that she can get her share of the bridewealth. If the divorce happens before the son-in-law has paid all *danga* that entitles him to the children, the father-in-law can negotiate to retain some of the bridewealth paid for the granddaughters that grow under his care. If the children that the mother brings to her people at divorce are boys, most of these would go back to their father, even if he would have refused to pay for their upkeep during their stay with their mother's people. It makes a man feel good to be able to live among his father's people. In his maternal grandfather's home, the grandson is referred to as *mwana wemukwasha*, which literally means, son of the son-in-law, and it sounds derogatory.

The modern civil law of Zimbabwe demands that children that are under the age of eighteen at the time of divorce should be supported by the father, and failure to do that can land the defaulter in jail. Again, the custody of children can be given to the mother, but it is generally believed that the children belong to the father, and should stay with him. Many women may not try to fight for the custody of children in modern courts of law unless the children are still too young to stay with their father. This understanding gives the divorced mother an opportunity to remarry without worrying about what to do with the children. Although some stepfathers can take care of their stepchildren, most Shona men resent doing that. A stepchild is referred to as *mubvandiripo*, which is a derogatory term meaning the child

---

29. Bullock, *The Mashona*, 367.
30. Bullock, *Mashona Laws and Customs*, 42.
31. Bullock, *The Mashona*, 368–69.

who came with the mother. Another insulting term that is sometimes used for a stepchild is *gora* (wild cat).

Let us revisit the principal parts of every rite of passage. The bride is concealed to the outsiders using the cloth with which she covers herself. The crisis periods she must undergo are her separation from family of birth, and the covering of her face when she enters the homestead of her husband. The cloth distinguishes her from the rest of the people present. The time of crisis can also refer to that period before her first pregnancy, a period in which the permanence of her marriage is not yet decided. The longer it takes for the woman to become pregnant, the worse the crisis period. The period of revelation happens every time the bride takes off her veil from her face so that the husband's relatives can see it. It also refers to the moment it becomes clearly visible that the wife is pregnant. Every time the bride removes the veil from her face, there is much jubilation and ululation. In the traditional past, a celebration called *mutimba* was thrown for the bride at the onset of marriage.

The incorporation of the new wife takes some time. This woman would have been born and bred in a completely different family. She should unlearn some of the family values she would have learnt from her family of origin, and learn the values of her new family. This unlearning and re-learning of values is the most difficult part of marriage, and sometimes the *muroora* is found wanting in one way or the other. In the past, the *muroora* was supposed to live and work in her mother-in-law's kitchen for more than a year. She had to prepare meals and do the laundry for all the husband's brothers and sisters that were still living with their mother. It was not until after the mother-in-law felt that the time had arrived to give the new wife her own kitchen, which is known as *kutegeswa*, when the *muroora* had to move into her own place. The word *kutegeswa* has the connotations of setting up the stones *(mapfihwa)* that balance the pot when cooking. No *muroora* can just get out of her mother-in-law's kitchen, and start her own cooking unless the *kutegeswa* ritual is performed. Even after *kutegeswa*, the *muroora* is expected to give the father-in-law some food, at least once every day, and it is known as *gunere*.

The new wife is also initiated into the family secrets of her husband's family that she should not share with outsiders. The *varoora* who gossip about their new families' secrets are accused of gossiping (*makuhwa*), and may be disciplined for that. However, it should be noted that the woman's incorporation into the family of her husband is not complete, for she remains an outsider among her husband's people. She may be excluded in the family rituals that the members of her husband's family undertake. She is referred to as *mutogwa*, which means outsider. When she dies, she is buried at her husband's home, but her family of origin should preside over her burial. They are responsible for cutting her waist band called *mutimwi*, and the disposal of her *chinu*, which is a container in which the traditional sacred body lotion was kept. They may also dispose of her underwears. If the burial rituals are not performed meticulously, the deceased woman's spirit may come back as an avenging spirit to punish the relatives of her husband, including her own children. So, the incorporation of the Shona woman into her husband's family is partial.

Death Rites

In most cultures and religious traditions of the world, "Death is a very solemn event fraught with danger for both the deceased and the living; hence, precaution must be taken to ensure that everything is done properly."[32] Although some Africans believe that death is not the end to one's life because a person's spirit continues to live as an ancestor, death still terrifies them. Death reminds most people of their limitedness and finitude. In the past, among the Shona, death was so devastating that children were not allowed to attend funerals unless the deceased was a close family member. This exclusion of children was intended to cushion them from experiencing the limitedness and frailty of humanity. Although most people spend all their time evading death, everyone knows that sooner or later, it will catch up with them, and when that moment comes, there is nothing that a person can do to escape. What terrifies most people is the lack of knowledge of what happens after death. Consequently, the dead must be accorded meticulous burial rites to give them the best chances in the next life, whatever its nature, and to prevent their offended spirits from coming back to haunt their living relatives.

Among the Shona, as soon as it is realized that someone is going to die at home, a close relative should watch him all the time. Usually, it is the duty of the women to keep watch and care for the terminally ill. As soon as the sick person dies, the family member who is present should immediately close the dying person's eyes and mouth before the body becomes rigid. The deceased's arms should be folded so that they are not scattered about. In the past, the legs of the dead person were supposed to be folded as well. This folding of the legs was beneficial to the grave diggers because the length and width of the pit would be determined by the length and width of the corpse. The folding of the dead body produced the shape of an unborn baby in its mother's womb. The grave signified the woman's womb in which the spirit of the dead person would wait until the performance of the cleansing

32. Imasogie, *African Traditional Religion*, 62.

ceremony that would initiate the dead into ancestorhood. Nowadays, the legs are not folded since most people are buried in coffins that fit the length of the body. Most of these preliminary rituals are now performed by those medical people who are present when a person dies at the hospital. The rituals may also be performed by the morticians who may apply a little make-up to the deceased to make him or her look presentable.

As soon as it is confirmed that the sick person has died, those around, particularly women, should cry out loudly (*mariro*). Any woman who fails to wail might be accused of being hard-hearted, or worse still, a witch. This crying alerts other villagers as to the demise of the sick person whose sickness they are aware of and they immediately rush to the home of the deceased person to perform the ritual of *kubata mavoko*, which literally means, to hold hands. Each villager greets every mourner who would have arrived before him, and says, "*Nedzoyi/Nedzinoparadza/Nematambudziko*," to which the one being greeted should answer, "*Awonokwa*." *Matambudziko* is a Shona word for suffering, and *awonekwa*, may be translated to mean, "we have experienced suffering." Although Shona men are not forbidden to cry loudly, it is considered unmanly for them to do that. Men should be strong. Of course, they may shed tears quietly.

If a person dies at a place far away from home, for instance, in town, his body should spend at least one night at the home where the burial rites will be carried out. Ordinarily, the kitchen, which is the sacred place for most Shona people, is preferred. Women do the watch over the body, while singing and dancing in the house in which the body is. Usually, Christian songs are sung even if the dead person was not a Christian. Sometimes, secular and Christian songs are mixed during the watch. Men may come in and out of the watch room as they please, but their ordinary place is outside, where they may spend the night around a fire. Some men may drink beer to down their sorrows. During the night, all burial arrangements are made so that the burial rites may be completed the following morning. Before burial, the body of the dead must be bathed and clothed in clean clothes. The bath does not need to be a wet bath, so a wet towel can be used to clean all the body parts that easily accumulate sweat, particularly, armpits, private parts, mouth, eyes, and anus. Usually close male relatives bath the corpse of men, and female relatives do the same for women. Both the towel and water used are buried with the body. If the person is a converted Christian, she may be dressed and buried in her Christian guild regalia, which is common among African Christians.

Early in the morning of the burial, a close relative of the dead should mark the grave, which the Shona call *kutema ruhahu*. Among the Korekore people of Zimbabwe, *ruhahu* is marked by the oldest grandson from the dead man's sisters or a close friend *(sahwira)* of the deceased.[33] If the dead person is a woman, *ruhahu* must be marked by a member of her family of origin. Once the first mark is made, other people may start digging the grave. Usually, only men do the digging while woman are keeping watch over the body, and cooking the food that will be consumed by the mourners. If the dead person is a Christian, the pastor may lead his rituals at that time, although some Christian rituals may run concurrently with the traditional ones. When the grave is ready, the body is taken out of the house on a stretcher called *bwanyanza,* or in a coffin, and is carried to the grave site by close relatives. The pall bearers place the coffin on the ground for three times before arriving at the grave to allow the spirit of the dead to rest. Women, particularly, *varoora,* who walk in front of the pall bearers, may sweep the path to the grave ahead of the coffin. They also carry the water pots and tins to the grave, and they should be offered a gift before they can place the water pitchers by the graveside. Some of them may also spread their cloths known as *zambias* on the path to the grave, so that the coffin can be placed on top of them during the resting times. Some Shona groups make sure that the corpse faces a certain direction. Some food and utensils might be put in the grave after the coffin has been lowered, for future consumption by the dead.

If the dead person was not married, some rituals to ensure that his spirit does not seek recognition as an ancestor are performed. The spirit of an unmarried person may wander among aliens where it can be accepted as an alien spirit *(shavi).* The close relatives of the dead person must cast the first lumps of soil into the grave, and then the rest of the people do likewise. As soon as the grave is completely covered with soil, all the people present may gather rocks from the vicinity. Only one rock, per person, at a time is allowed. Usually the top of the grave is completely covered by rocks, with the head rock standing taller than all other rocks. Once the burial is done, all the men who would have participated in the digging and covering of the grave may wash their hands, and the remaining water is sprinkled around the grave after which no one may step on that ground. If witches disturb the grave over the night, their footprints would be seen, and might be identified by other villagers. In the past, when most people did not have shoes, villagers could easily identify fellow villagers by their footprints. It should be noted that the burial should not be done during mid-day, particularly, between noon and 3:00 pm.

Among the Shona, the close relatives of the deceased may shave their hair after burial, and may not shave the new hair until after the cleansing ceremony *(kurova guva/kugadzira).* The Shona word *kurova* means to beat,

---

33. Gelfand, *Shona Religion with Special Reference to the Makorekore,* 121.

and *guva*, means grave. The word *kugadzira*, that is mostly used by the Karanga of Masvingo for this process means to make or produce. In this case, it refers to the making of an ancestor. If the performance of the ceremony is delayed, the mourners may shave their hair about six months after the burial. The closest female relative of the dead person wears black dresses or veils to indicate that she is mourning. Men may pin a black piece of cloth unto their shirts, if they are mourning. The black color signifies the darkness that death brings to the family.

Traditionally, all joyous celebrations such as weddings were supposed to be postponed, if a close family member had died. The phrase used for such a situation is *musha mutema*, which can be translated as, the home is dark. Those members of the family who are unable to attend the funeral may come later, since they are required to do *kubata maoko*, which means to convey their condolences by shaking the hands of the close relatives of the dead, who would have been present at his burial. They are also supposed to go to the grave to place a small rock on it while introducing themselves to the dead by name and relationship. The Shona call this ritual, *kukanda chibwe*, meaning placing the small rock on the grave. This *kukanda chibwe* ritual signifies the solidarity between those who would have buried the dead and the one who was absent. Those family members who refuse to perform the *kukanda chibwe* ritual aggravate the spirit of the dead. The family members that are not on talking terms with the deceased should forgive him when he dies because *wafa wanaka* (the one who has died becomes upright). It is not good for anyone to hold a grudge against a family member that has died.

Some Shona groups slaughter a cow or goat to be consumed by the mourners, and they call it, *nhevedzo*. Usually, the food is eaten after the burial, although nothing stops people from eating earlier, if the food is ready. The Karanga have what they call *mahakurimwi*, which refer to the avoidance of working in the fields after burying someone. Ordinarily, the duration is supposed to be one week, but it may be shortened due to the season in which the death takes place. During the rainy season, *mahakurimwi* may be shortened to three days. On the day of burial, most people announce the date of the *nyaradzo*, which is a Christian ritual that is performed to pray for the soul of the dead, and to commiserate with the mourners. At almost the same time, the Karanga hold a ritual known as *masuka foshora*, which refers to the cleaning of the shovels of those who would have dug the grave. Beer is brewed and a goat may be slaughtered at this ceremony. Some Shona people may consult a traditional medical practitioner concerning the cause of the death of the deceased. This consultation is called *gata*. But if the deceased was advanced in age, most people may not perform the *gata*. Other Shona groups delay the *gata* until a few weeks or days before the cleansing ceremony. The last big ritual is the cleansing ceremony (*kurova guva*) that is intended to bring back into the family the spirit of the dead as an ancestor.[34]

There are no mourning rituals for still-born and premature babies who die at birth. The burial rituals are avoided to fool the witches and evil spirits who want to see the mother suffer. There is no official *kubata mavoko* that is done for such babies. Their bodies are buried in the river bank, at the edge of the water to cool them. If the baby is still a fetus, it is placed in a clay pot and buried in the river bank.[35] Only old women, who have reached menopause may attend such burial rituals, for it is believed that if a woman of child-bearing age attends, the spirit of the baby might cause the deaths of her future babies. If the misfortune happens at the hospital, the fetus is cremated as per the policy of the hospital.

Christianity and Shona Rites of Passage

The coming of Christianity to Africa, and its reluctant and gradual acceptance by most Africans challenged most indigenous rites of passage. The early Christian missionaries demonized African birth rituals by laughing at them as superstitious. The construction of hospitals has significantly transformed most of the traditional birth rituals. The traditional midwives have been replaced by the nurses and gynecologists at the hospital, where most women give birth. Hospitals may dispose of the placenta in accordance with the policy of the hospital. Although some hospitals may allow the family of the birthing mother to keep the placenta, in most cases, it is difficult for the family to keep the placenta fresh, from the time of birth until they reach their rural home to bury it. Hence, most Shona mothers allow the hospital staff to dispose of it accordingly.

Christianity has also affected the names that people give to their children. Missionaries gave names of saints to their followers' children because their indigenous names were considered evil. Nowadays, when a child is born, some Christians take that child to be blessed or even baptized by their priest at their local church. Medals of saints may be given to the child, and holy water sprinkled over him to protect him from evil spirits. However, some Shona people show religious allegiance to both Christianity and the traditional religion by soliciting the assistance of both Christian and traditional blessings and protection for the child. Before the children are presented to the church for baptism or blessing, they are traditionally

---

34. The ritual of *kurova guva* will be explored in detail in chapter 4 of this book.
35. Gelfand, *Shona Religion with Special Reference to the Makorekore*, 124.

immunized for fontanelle *(nhova)* and other childhood ailments. Sometimes a Shona child has both a saint's medal and the traditional necklace *(zango)*. Some parents who want to appear more Christian may take their newly born babies to the members of the African Independent Churches, who practice both Christian and traditional immunization of the *nhova*. Evidently, some Shona Christians perform both traditional and Christian rituals for the protection of their children from evil spirits and people.

The traditional circumcision of young men by some African ethnic groups has been criticized as barbaric and unhygienic. Several Christian churches discourage young men from participating in such rituals by introducing many Christian youth programs to take care of their needs. Clitoridectomy has been outlawed in many African countries as the genital mutilation of women. The Karanga rituals of the sausage tree have disappeared. The traditional testing of boys for fertility is gone. However, the church has failed to stop girls from receiving the traditional pubertal instructions concerning their marital and adult responsibilities. There are still a few ethnic groups that test their girls for virginity, and shame those that are found wanting. Circumcision for boys has continued unabated in many African countries, although some leaders now encourage the sacred practitioners of that ritual to follow modern hygienic methods. It seems that many Africans still hold on to their traditional rites of passage. The same boys that are baptized in the Christian churches also perform their traditional rites of passage in their villages. Some Africans feel that either Christian or African rituals alone are not adequate, hence, they want to benefit from both religious traditions.

Most traditional marriage rites of passage have remained intact. Bridewealth is still mandatory even though many Africans have accepted the Christian wedding as the norm. Some young men and women preparing for marriage receive instructions from both Christian and traditional sacred practitioners. Among the Shona, the traditional marriage rituals precede the Christian wedding. The bridewealth negotiations and other marital rituals must be done first before the couple can marry in church. The Roman Catholic Church teaches that for a marriage to be valid the marital consents must be free from any defect and should be exchanged before three witnesses, one of whom should be the official witness or assistant of the church, usually a priest, deacon, or bishop.[36] Marriage is sacramental if contracted by two baptized persons, and is indissoluble once ratified, and consummated through the normal human sexual act. The purpose of marriage is for the establishment of a "community of life and love" for the "good of the

---

36. Haffner, *The Sacramental Mystery*, 278–82.

spouses and for the procreation and education of children."[37] In the Roman Catholic Church, failure to conceive is not a cause for the annulment of the marriage. Marriage can only be annulled if it is discovered that it was never validly contracted right from its beginning, due to some diriment impediment that existed at the time of its contraction. It can also be dissolved if either party's consent was defective. Other issues such as antecedent and perpetual impotency, altered mental state of one of the spouses, deceit, the incarceration of one of the spouses, among other issues, may be grounds for the dissolution of a Catholic marriage.

For the Shona, marriage is both a family and communal celebration that should be contracted in the presence of the families and relatives of those who are marrying. The couple does not exchange any vows because the offer of bridewealth by the wife-receivers, and its reception by the wife-givers give evidence of the couple's consents to marry. The Shona marriage is dissoluble. The consummation of the marriage is gradual, and is confirmed by the birth of enough children. If there are no children in a marriage, it becomes shaky, and may be dissolved. Bridewealth is crucial, and all men, including Christians should pay their bridewealth. For most Christians, the payment of bridewealth is contradictory to the tenets of Christianity, yet they still pay it. Marriage is another area in which both the traditional and Christian rituals run concurrently, or one immediately after the other. Although early missionaries tried to abolish the payment of bridewealth, it has survived up to now, and there is no sign that it will disappear soon.

The missionaries almost succeeded in stamping out polygamy. Among many African ethnic groups, the practice is almost gone. However, the missionaries' endeavor to eradicate polygamy has received a terrible blow from some African Independent Churches that allow polygamous marriages. It seems that when Africans felt that they could not perform dual religious rites, they pulled out of the mainline churches to establish their own churches that allowed them to integrate traditional and Christian rites of passage. In Zimbabwe, those men who would want to marry more than one wife, may also use the Customary Marriages Act [Chapter 5:07] that allows them to do that.

The Shona death rituals have also caused much division among Christians. When someone is sick, Christians may summon their leader to pray for him. Roman Catholics take it a step further by offering the sacrament of the sick in which the sick person is anointed with sacred oil. The rosary may be recited on the night before the burial. Mass may be celebrated before or during the funeral, and the corpse may be blessed with holy water. The

---

37. Martin de Agar, *A Handbook on Canon Law*, 2nd ed., 199.

Shona still perform the traditional rituals of death if someone dies at home as explained above. The priest may be invited if the deceased is a Christian, but that does not stop the people from performing the traditional burial rituals. Usually, the traditional and Christian rituals run side by side. The traditional sacred practitioners run the show, and the priest is only invited to perform his part whenever necessary.

The early missionaries tried to ban the cleansing ceremony to no avail. The Roman Catholic Church ended up instituting an inculturated burial ritual, after having failed to ban *kurova guva* for many years. In 1978, the Catholic Bishops in Zimbabwe approved a modified ritual of the dead (*kuchenura munhu*), which received the Vatican's approval on an experimental basis in 1981.[38] For the Roman Catholic Church, the soul of the dead awaits the last judgment, or may go to heaven. The Shona people believe that the dead may become ancestors, and come back to their families to watch over them. The Shona have no equivalent of purgatory and hell. Their God does not punish anyone after death.

It is very interesting that the encounter between African Traditional Religion and Christianity has benefitted the Shona more in the sense of having dual religiosity. They benefit from both the Christian and traditional worldviews. Some of them try to fulfill both the traditional and Christian religious obligations. If they fail to get answers from the Christian God, they may turn to the God of their ancestors, who many Africans argue is the same God as the Christian God. In times of drought, they pray to both the Christian God, and the God of Matonjeni. If the God of their ancestors refuses to bless them, they may turn to the Christian God. Most of the time, they do not have to wait for an answer, for they try to appease both Gods at the same time. Although, some of them perform traditional rituals secretly, there are many who do them openly. Paradoxically, the coming of Christianity to Africa benefitted and affected Africans simultaneously. The African got the better part of the bargain. He who has acquired two ways of killing a cat stands a better chance of succeeding. When African Gods ignore them, Africans may solicit the help of the Christian Gods, and the other way around.

---

38. Creary, *Domesticating a Religious Import*, 222.

3

The Shona Concept of God

One of the primary tasks of the early Christian missionaries, anthropologists, and some colonial administrators in Africa was to explore the indigenous beliefs of the colonized people to determine the efficacy of such beliefs. The issue of whether God existed in Africa or not before the arrival of Christian missionaries was one of the most contentious issues under their microscope. Most of the missionaries who investigated the concept of God in Africa before the arrival of the Christian God erroneously concluded that Africans could not conceive of a deity, since God was too abstract and philosophical for the puny African minds. One of them, J. B. Danquah, is said to have argued that the Akan Supreme Being was a mere deified ancestor.[1] Consequently, the Akan and other African people were believed to worship ancestors instead of the one true God, an assertion that some African theologians such as John S. Mbiti vehemently rebut. Mbiti argues that although ancestors occupy a central position in the African cosmology they are not worshipped.[2]

What is interesting to note is that the early Western writers did not deny the fact that Africans had a God or Gods, but they tried to prove that the African God or Gods were inferior to the Christian God that they had brought from Europe. Although some of them were convinced of their findings, many of them might have pursued that line of argument to make their religion acceptable to the Africans. It would have made no sense to the Africans if the missionaries had affirmed that the African God was as good as the Christian God, because doing so would have undermined the missionaries' efforts to convert Africans to Christianity. The African God had to be declared incapable of bestowing blessings on, and bringing salvation to Africans, in order to persuade them to accept a superior God. Most Africans accepted the missionaries' message, though some of them did that reservedly.

---

1. Parrinder, *African Traditional Religion*, 31.
2. Mbiti, *African Religions and Philosophy*, 8.

Mwari and the Early Missionaries in Zimbabwe

The Christian missionaries who came to Zimbabwe in the nineteenth century were not different from their kith and kin who went to other African countries. Their primary goal was to win souls for Christ, which proved to be an insurmountable task in the early years of their evangelization as explained in chapter 1 of this book. When they arrived in Zimbabwe, both the Shona and Ndebele people had an elaborate belief in the Supreme God, who the Shona called Mwari, and the Ndebele, Umlimo. The Shona believed that Mwari was the creator of the universe and everything that is found in it.[3] Mwari was believed to be indifferent to individual needs, but was concerned with national issues such as the fertility of the land and rainmaking.[4] He was only consulted during periods of drought, through emissaries that were sent to his most holy residency, the Matonjeni cave in Matopos Hills, on the outskirts of the present-day city of Bulawayo. Later, Mwari assumed a political portfolio, and was influential in the Ndebele and Shona Uprisings (1896–98) against the British colonial rule.

At this point, let us explore the theories concerning the origins of Mwari, the God of Matonjeni. Most of the theories of the origin of the Shona concept of Mwari are based on the etymology of the term Mwari. The major challenge to those that have tried to investigate the origins of the Mwari worship is that the name itself does not sound Shona, because most Shona names have meanings, but Mwari does not seem to mean anything. One of the earliest theories is said to have come from Father Loubiere, SJ, who argues that the name Mwari is the *Shonarization* of the word Mwali, which has its origins among the Sena people of the Zambezi area, and refers to God. A similar term, *muwali,* is used by the same people to refer to the initiated women, which has led some scholars to argue that Mwari might have been the Goddess of fertility.[5] It has been argued that Mwari was more concerned about rainmaking, which made the land fecund, and that makes him a fertility God. In Shona symbolism, rain resembles the sperms, and the soil symbolizes the womb. The raining itself and the percolation of the water into the soil can be likened to the sexual act, which results in the germination and growing of the crops and fruits that sustain life.

The second theory says that Mwari might have originated from the area near Lake Kilimanjaro, and was brought to Zimbabwe by the Mbire people. Chief Nembire is believed to have travelled from Lake Tanganyika

---

3. Bhebe, *Christianity and Traditional Religion in Western Zimbabwe 1859–1923,* 19.
4. Thorpe, *African Traditional Religions,* 54.
5. Bullock, *The Mashona (The Indigenous Natives of S. Rhodesia),* 121.

at the beginning of the fourteenth century and resettled in the South.[6] The term *Muali* is used in that area to refer to God, the Sower, who is almost like the God of fertility. Daneel thinks that there is a striking affinity between *Muali* and Mwari, particularly his concern for the fertility of both crops and women.[7]

The other theory is said to be supported by Father Ignatious Chidavaenzi, a Zimbabwean biblical scholar. He believes that the name Mwari comes from the Shona word *muwari*, which is a noun that comes from the verb *kuwara*. *Kuwara* means to spread, and this portrays God as the creator.[8] Although this argument sounds attractive, it seems far-fetched because *kuwara* is usually associated with the spreading of the sleeping mat and blanket before people go to bed. Therefore, the word might not have the connotations of creation unless the sleeping mat is being spread for the purpose of sexual activities, which might not be the case in most *kuwara*.

The fourth theory says that the name Mwari is a contraction of the word *muari*, which refers to the irregular verb *to be*, and the word *muari* can be translated as "the one who is."[9] Some scholars have rejected this theory for its likeness to the biblical story of Moses and the burning bush that is found in the book of Genesis. It seems that the theory is an attempt to Christianize the Shona God to make him more acceptable to Christian missionaries.

The truth of the issue is that it is difficult to reconstruct a credible theory concerning the origins of the term Mwari. The greatest consolation that scholars of traditional religions of Africa do have is that there is no doubt that Mwari was the God of the Shona people. There is also consensus that Mwari's headquarters were at Matopos Hills, near the present-day city of Bulawayo. It is on the same hills where Cecil John Rhodes' tomb is located. There is also general agreement that Mwari was concerned with national issues, and was contacted on special occasions.[10] The messengers who visited Mwari's shrine never saw the face of Mwari, but only heard his voice that came from the cave. It was the responsibility of his priests to interpret his words. The voice is believed to have been coming from the high priest who impersonated Mwari, while the other priests—whose main responsibility was to translate the message for the benefit of the visitors—would sit with the enquirers by the sacred cave entrance, facing the East.[11] The visitors would enquire about

6. Daneel, *The God of the Matopos Hills*, 15–16.
7. Ibid., 16.
8. Creary, *Domesticating a Religious Import*, 204.
9. Ibid., 204.
10. Gelfand, *The African Witch*, 20.
11. Bhebe, *Christianity and Traditional Religion in Western Zimbabwe 1859–1923*, 19.

the challenges bedeviling their local communities, particularly drought. The voice would then identify the source of the problem, and how it could be remedied to enable the rain to come. Some people believe that as soon as the enquirers went back to their communities, and meticulously implemented the guidelines given to them by God, the rain would come. However, there were years when Mwari would not relent by giving people the rain that they would have asked for, and the people never lost trust in his magnanimity. They continued to hope that the following year God would forgive their transgressions, and grant them rain.

Some sacred men (*hosana*) and virgin women (*mbonga*) were dedicated to the service of Mwari at Matonjeni. This dedication would end when they got married. The *mbonga* cleaned the shrine premises, tended the land, sang, and danced in honor of God, and could become spirit mediums after marriage.[12] These women would have been brought to the shrine by their parents and offered to the high priest so that they could serve Mwari. The *hosana* also assisted in tending the land and sacred dancing during the annual rainmaking ceremony. Some of them were the messengers of Mwari to the different districts of the country. Both the *mbonga* and the *hosanas* were required to attend the annual rainmaking ceremony at the shrine. The *hosanas* were hosts of the *jukwa* spirits that are believed to have emanated from Mwari, and were responsible for rainmaking. Among various Shona groups, there were other men who were not *hosanas* but hosted the *jukwa* spirits. Most of them would be sent to Matonjeni by their communities whenever the rain had delayed. They too presided over the rain making ceremony (*mutoro/mukwerere*) as representatives of Mwari. As I was growing up in Nyajena, Masvingo, a well-respected *jukwa* spirit medium was Mr. Nhikiras Chapingura, who played a crucial role as a messenger to Matonjeni and at *mutoro* rituals.

Praise Names of Mwari

Mwari was also referred to using several praise names that came out of the Shona people's experiences of him.[13] The messengers who were sent to Matonjeni, after having eaten food, would remove their shoes, and sit with their backs to the cave entrance, and would clap their hands as a sacred greeting to

---

12. Daneel, *The God of the Matopos Hills*, 49–50.

13. Mwari has no gender and the Shona pronoun *iye* does not indicate the gender of the person being referred to. The pronoun *he* is used for convenience's sake, and not to downplay the possibility that Mwari could as well be a woman.

Mwari, while mentioning his praise names.[14] *Dzivaguru* was one of the most popular praise names used for Mwari. *Dzivaguru* is a compound word that comes from two Shona words, *dziva*, which means pool, and *guru*, which means big. Hence, *Dzivaguru* means the big pool. This name was a result of the Shona's reflection on the rain-giving character of God. They had experienced rain, year after year, and it seemed that the source of that rain was so big that it produced sufficient rain for everyone. The Shona believed that drought was not a result of the shortage of rain from its heavenly source, but a consequence of God's withholding of it, to compel the transgressors of the moral standards of the community to reform. The Shona might have had an idea of the ocean, which never runs dry. The name *Dzivaguru* was closely connected to *Chidziva Chepo*, meaning a small pool that has no beginning or end and never runs dry. The most popular Matonjeni cave was called *Mabweadziva*, meaning the stones of the pool.[15]

God was also referred to as *Musiki*, which means creator. Most Shona people still use this name to refer to God. This name was an acknowledgment of God's creative powers, after the Shona reflected on all his creation, particularly the rain that made the land fruitful. In their cosmogonic myths, the Shona stress that God is the creator of human beings, the universe, and everything that is in it. The *Mwedzi* creation story explains how the world, human beings, plants, and animals were created. The crux of the story is that Mwari created Mwedzi in the bottom of a pool. He then created Masasi (woman), Mwedzi's first temporary companion, who became the mother of all trees, grass, and bushes after being touched by the finger of Mwedzi that had been dipped in his medicinal horn. When Masasi's time with Mwedzi expired, she was replaced by another woman, Murongo, who became the mother of all animals and human beings. Murongo had a secret and illicit affair with the snake, which lived under their matrimonial bed. Because the snake sexually satisfied her, she gave her husband permission to sleep with his daughters, which resulted in the multiplication of human beings. Mwedzi was later bitten by Murongo's illicit lover, the snake, when he tried to force himself on her, and that resulted in a drought. Mwedzi's children were advised by the bones that they consulted to send Mwedzi back into the pool. They strangled him, and buried him together with Murongo, and then selected a new king.[16] The Mwedzi Cosmogonic myth is the Shona's acknowledgement of Mwari's creative character. The Shona also believe that the same Mwari continues to sustain the universe through the provi-

---

14. Daneel, *The God of the Matopo Hills*, 77.
15. Daneel, *Old and New in Southern Shona Independent Churches Vol. 1*, 81.
16. Bucher, *Spirits and Power*, 72.

sion of the rain that makes the land fertile. Connected to the praise name Musiki, is Musikavanhu, which means the creator of human beings. The name Musikavanhu emphasizes the centrality of human beings in God's creation. Everything was created to nourish and sustain human beings, but should be used with respect.

Nyadenga and *Wedenga*, which mean the owner of the sky, are variations of the same name for God. Although the epiphany of God was evidently experienced at Matonjeni, the Shona believed that the same God was the owner of the sky. His ownership of the sky was evidenced by the three wonders that they saw in the sky—the moon, sun, and the stars. The East (*mabvazuva*), from where the sun rises every day, was considered sacred. The visitors who were sent to the shrine of God had to sit with their backs to the entrance of the cave, while facing the East. The appearance of the new moon was a cause for celebration for both the Ndebele and Shona people. It signified a new beginning, and its crescent shape revealed the fortunes or misfortunes that the new month had in store for the people. The Shona's creation myth uses *Mwedzi* (Moon) as the name of the first person to be created. Monthly periods are called *kuenda kumwedzi*, which literally means going to the moon. This imaginary journey to the moon that happens every month, makes women not only powerful, but also extremely dangerous, spiritually. Consequently, Shona men are discouraged from being intimate with women during their imaginary trip to the moon, fearing that men could be weakened or even harmed. Such women were not allowed to actively assist in the ancestral rituals because their flow of blood would weaken the sacred practitioners, which was likely to invalidate the ritual. The Shona also believed that the two human-like shapes that are seen on the full moon were human beings who had been punished for working on the ancestral sacred day of resting (*chisi*).

In the sky, the Shona also saw the stars of which two, *Masasi* (morning star) and *Murongo* (evening star), were sacred. In the *Mwedzi* cosmogonic myth, *Masasi* and *Murongo* are the names of the first women to be created, and the mothers of human beings and everything that is in the world. In addition to that, the rains come down from the sky, which makes it the source of life. It is also in the sky where God shows his unparalleled might through lightning and thunderstorms, which can be hazardous to humanity, particularly those people who have secretly violated the laws of the land. Some Shona groups perform a ritual whenever there are lightning and thunderstorms. My grandmother would insert the two cooking sticks (*musika nemugoti*) in the water container (*chirongo*) to neutralize the effects of the lightning. Although she did not tell us why she thought that the ritual would spare us from lightning strikes, it seems that the ritual symbolized the sexual act between the life-giving forces of water and the cooking sticks, and that might have pacified the angry spirits. The lightning also fertilizes the land by breaking atmospheric nitrogen atoms and creating nitrogen oxides, which then dissolve to form nitrates that are carried to the soil through the rain. Although the Shona might not have been aware of this complicated process, they knew from their experiences that lightning was good for the plants.

The Shona also call God *Samasimba*, which means the one who wields power. They experience God's power in rain, lightning, and other forces of nature. His power is also experienced in the birth, growth, and death of all animals, plants, and people. Although human beings have a hand in the procreation of other people, only God tends to their growth and health until he finally allows them to die. The power of God is also witnessed through the mysterious ways in which he created the first human beings. Connected to *Samasimba* is *Chirazazamauya*, which means, the giver of blessings. The Shona believe that all blessings come from God through the ancestors. For them, the three greatest blessings from God are good health, longevity, and prosperity. It should be noted that the Shona still use these praise names to refer to God.

Mwari and Ancestors

The relationship between Mwari and ancestors was very clear to the Shona. They were both spirits, but God was the Supreme Being, who sat on top of the hierarchical pyramid. The ancestors derived their power and authority from God. Mwari was different from ancestors in that he was never a human being like ancestors. He had no beginning and no end. Mwari was the creator of the universe and all that is in it. At Matonjeni, what visitors heard was the voice of God through the high priest, and the Shona knew that the high priest was not Mwari. The praise names that have been explored above were only used for Mwari, and not for ancestors. Ancestors were the ministers of God, who took care of every day needs of their living family members, but God was concerned about those issues that were beyond the jurisdiction of the ancestors. The God of Matonjeni was good at delegating responsibilities to the ancestors, hence, he had ample time to address national problems.

The Encounter between Mwari Worship and Christianity

When the early missionaries arrived in Zimbabwe, in the nineteenth century, they did not quite understand Mwari's nature and operations. Thomas Morgen Thomas, a missionary of the London Missionary Society, mistook Mwari's high priest for Mwari himself. He describes Ukwali (Mwari) as a one-footed man, believed to be "mighty and greedy," dwelling under one of their mountains in a cave, and argues that: "In reality, however, he is no other than one of the original aristocrats of the country, who being well versed in the traditions of his forefathers, the priestcraft and witchcraft of his tribe, manages to blind the people and hide his true character from them."[17] He further argues that Ukwali's knowledge and wisdom was a result of the conniving between the high priest and the people who lived in the shrine village. For Thomas Morgan Thomas, Mwari was a fake God, and not worthy of being worshipped.

Some scholars have also argued that the early missionaries were bent on desecrating the Mwari shrine as soon as they arrived. For instance, the colonial administrators of Zimbabwe had the audacity to bury Cecil John Rhodes—the leader of the British South Africa Company that colonized Zimbabwe—on the Matopos Hills, and by so doing desecrating the sacred home of God. They challenged the efficacy of the rainmaking ceremonies, and later forbade the Shona Christians from attending them. For many years, the use of the name Mwari, with reference to the Christian God, was forbidden by the missionaries.[18] During the Anglo-Ndebele War (1893–94), the Mwari high priest, priests, priestesses, *hosanas*, and *mbonga* were unceremoniously driven away from the sacred caves.

Was the Christian God very different from the Mwari? A closer look at the God of Matonjeni and the expatriate God brought by the missionaries may identify many similarities between the two. Both Gods were almighty, eternal, monotheistic, and creators of the universe and all that is in it. Both Gods had priests, priestesses, deacons, and deaconesses who were intermediaries between them and the people. Both Gods had voices or messengers that they used to make known their wills to the people. They were also the Supreme Beings in the hierarchy of spirituals beings. Both Gods were incorporeal. It is interesting to note that both Gods could be aggravated by the transgressions of the laws of the land by some people. Both had shrines from which they could communicate to their followers. Both Gods satisfactorily

---

17. Thomas, *Eleven Years in Central South Africa*, 288.
18. Creary, *Domesticating a Religious Import*, 246.

provided for the needs of their followers. Consequently, some theologians have argued that Mwari, the God of the Shona, and the God of Christians were indeed the *same* God.

However, the two Gods had differences too. The God of the missionaries involved himself in both national *and individual* issues, unlike the Shona God, who only concerned himself with national issues, and delegated his authority to the ancestors to deal with family and personal issues. The missionaries' God was explicitly mentioned in almost every ritual that they performed, but Mwari had very few rituals directed to him. His name was not even mentioned in most rituals that were performed for ancestors. There existed a disagreement among the Christian missionaries concerning the nature of their God. Consequently, the London Missionary Society and Jesuits had different, and sometimes conflicting views of their God, yet the Shona God was homogenous and spoke with one voice. Mwari did not send his messengers to convert any other people to the Shona religion, yet the missionaries claimed that their God wished to convert the whole world to Christianity. The Shona God did not undermine and demean the Gods of other people in the same way the missionaries attacked all other Gods except their own. The Christian God undermined other Gods by sending his messengers to impose his worship on the people who already worshipped their own Gods, but Mwari only cared for his own people.

The question that might be asked at this juncture is whether the missionaries managed to obliterate the God of Matonjeni or not. The answer to this question is yes and no. They did destroy the worship of Mwari to a certain extent. They desecrated the Matonjeni shrines, and harassed the priests, *mbonga*, and *hosanna* of Mwari. They discouraged the Shona from holding the annual rainmaking ceremonies at Matonjeni, and most communities stopped sending their messengers to Matonjeni to inquire about national issues. They belittled the God of Matonjeni as a fake and ineffective God. Eventually, the Shona were completely prevented from worshipping Mwari at Matonjeni.

However, it can also be argued that the missionaries failed to destroy the God of Matonjeni. The God of Matonjeni's official name, Mwari, has become the official Shona name for the Christian God in Zimbabwe. The rainmaking ceremonies (*mutoro/mukwerere*) are still being performed in most Shona villages every year. The praise names of Mwari, such as *Musiki, Musikavanhu, Nyadenga, Samasimba*, and others, have found their way into the Christian sacred and liturgical writings. Yes, the missionaries may have succeeded in desecrating and chasing Mwari away from his official residence at Matonjeni, but by so doing, they decentralized his presence to all the districts of Zimbabwe. The banishment of Mwari from Matonjeni was a blessing in disguise because it compelled him to become a personal God who could be approached directly by everyone.

It can also be argued that the missionaries later realized that there was no difference between Mwari of Matonjeni and the God that they claimed to have brought from Europe. The way some Zimbabweans partake in both Christian and traditional rituals may be an indication that the Mwari of Matonjeni might have faked his death by clothing himself in Christian garments, for the sake of his survival. His spirit can be seen in some Shona cultural practices' resilience despite the demonization that they continue to receive at the hands of Christian evangelists. Although Mwari's holy caves at Matopos Hills have been irrevocably violated and desecrated, and his priesthood and diaconate banished by the Europeans, he has found himself a better dwelling place in the churches that the missionaries have built throughout Zimbabwe. He continues to speak to his people through the Christian bishops, priests, nuns, pastors, apostles, and prophets. Probably one day, the Shona people will retrace the footprints of their ancestors back to Matonjeni, just like the Jewish people were able to go back to Jerusalem to worship their God at the Wailing Wall.

4

The Centrality of Ancestors

It is difficult to pinpoint the purpose for which human beings were created, but we know the aspirations, hopes, and fears that they have. They want to live a happy, healthy, and long life. In fact, if it were their decision to make, human beings would opt for an everlasting life that is free from all suffering, pain, struggles, imperfections, sorrows, and toils. The impossibility of the attainment of such a life continues to disappoint humanity. It is painful to realize that life entails suffering, sickness, imperfections, and finitude. There is no warranted length of life here on earth because death comes to everyone, and at times, untimely. Some people die before they even see the light of the sun. Some die young, before they experience what it means to be human. Some die in middle ages, leaving offspring without anyone to protect and provide for them. Some people die of accidents, and others of natural causes. Some die violently, and others die peacefully. Death is like a bridge between two islands through which everyone must cross over. The only consolation humanity has is that those who are strong and lucky may live to see their grandchildren and great grandchildren.

Although human beings are individuals, each with her own friends and enemies, death remains the commonest enemy that all human beings must face. The biggest challenge surrounding death is the absence of some concrete knowledge about what happens to the human soul after it leaves the human body. Most human beings have refused to accept the notion that death is the end of human life, and that there is nothing but the skeleton after death. Religious traditions have become handy in trying to give humanity the hope of an everlasting life. Although some religions claim that there is only one life—this present life, and that death marks the end of one's life, most religious traditions disagree with that notion. Most religious traditions do provide insights into how life after death might look. Likewise, African Traditional Religion teaches that death is not the end of human life, but a transition from one form of life to another. Those who die will continue to live as ancestors (*midzimu*), or any one form of the numerous spirits that fill the universe.

Ancestors are the dead paternal and maternal relatives that are invited back into the family as spiritual members, so that they may protect, intercede for, and bless their living family members. John S. Mbiti has paradoxically named them "the living dead."[1] Ancestors are living in the sense that they are still concerned with the affairs of their living relatives. Although they cannot be seen by human eyes, and touched by human hands, they are ever present in the homes of their relatives, and participate in family activities. Some family members offer portions of food and drinks to the ancestors as an acknowledgement of their presence, and an act of hospitality. Ancestors also live in the memories of their living relatives. Some family members still have the ancestors' pictures, either on paper or in their memories. Some people offer them flowers and libation during memorial days. The Shona believe that ancestors are ever present wherever their living relatives are. Some people give their children names of their living or dead parents and grandparents as a reminder of their continual existence.

Ancestors are also dead because they no longer possess physical bodies. Their bodies stopped breathing, and were either buried or cremated. They now live in the spiritual form, which is not limited by space or time. They neither suffer nor die. They are always present, yet invisible. They have dual citizenship in the spiritual and physical worlds, and enjoy the benefits of both worlds. They have one leg in the world of the living and the other in the world of spirits, and perfectly understand both worlds. For John S. Mbiti, ancestors are bilingual, for they speak the languages of spirits and humans.[2]

Who Becomes an Ancestor?

Not every person who dies can become an ancestor because there are qualifications and disqualifications that are involved. The most critical qualification is that of having begotten children. Ordinarily, one of those children should be male. The belief is that one becomes an ancestor for the sole purpose of protecting and blessing one's offspring. The other reason that makes begetting of children crucial is the requirement for the cleansing ceremony that should be performed by the children of the deceased. No one can become an ancestor unless that ritual is performed. So, without children one dies forever. That makes marriage and the bearing of children crucial among the Shona. To deliberately refuse to bear children is not only an insult to oneself, but to the whole community. It is choosing death instead of life, and finitude of humanity, instead of perpetuity. Among the Shona, the most conventional way of begetting children is through marriage. However,

---

1. Mbiti, *African Religions and Philosophy*, 2nd ed., 81–82.
2. Ibid., 82.

it does not matter if the children are born out of wedlock or within a marriage, because they can still perform the cleansing ceremony without which the deceased person cannot become an ancestor. Unfortunately, adopted children cannot perform that cleansing ritual because they are not related to the dead person by *blood*.

Normally, the performance of the cleansing ceremony is the male children's responsibility. Be that as it may, female children can perform the ritual with the assistance of male relatives in the case where the deceased has no surviving son. Male children are crucial because one of them carries the name of the deceased father. In the case of the death of the mother, one of her granddaughters may inherit her name. However, the shouldering of the responsibility to perform the cleansing ceremony by the male children does not take anything away from female children because they can still be hosts of male ancestors, and become the sacred practitioners in their families of origin.

What happens if a couple fails to beget children? In the past, whenever that heart-rending challenge arose, the culprit was almost always thought to be the wife. She would be blamed or even divorced for that. Although in some childless marriages the husband was the culprit, it was inconceivable and shameful to imagine the man as having fertility problems. In the Shona society, to be a man is to be able to bear children, and very few men may admit that they are infertile. Traditionally, married men who failed to father children with their official wives would secretly try their luck outside the marriage in extramarital affairs. If the man succeeded in impregnating his mistress, he would feel vindicated, and would either keep his barren wife or divorce her. If the family of the husband discovered that their own son was infertile and could not impregnate his wife, arrangements would be made to enable the younger brother of the man to secretly bear children for his older brother with his brother's wife. Of course, the affair was not supposed to be a romantic one, but the performance of one's duty. In cases where there were no male children, some men married more than one wife just to make sure that one of them would give birth to a son. Begetting children is crucial, and whoever fails to bear them is doomed forever.

Longevity is another requirement, and it is understood in two different ways. First, it is understood in terms of numbers. One should have lived for a long time, and might have seen one's grandchildren or great grandchildren. A long life exposes one to numerous experiences, which are believed to make a person wiser and more knowledgeable. The person who has lived a long life would have contributed many things for the wellbeing of the community. Furthermore, old age takes one closer to the ancestors regarding seniority. The closer one is to the ancestors of the family, the wiser one is believed to be in matters of spirituality and the traditions of the family. Longevity is also understood in the sense of progeny that ensures the continuity of the family and clan name. Anyone who begets a child has already attained longevity. If he dies, he continues to live as an ancestor because his children would perform the cleansing ceremony (*kurova guva*) for his spirit. In fact, those who live a long life in terms of years, yet have no children, are technically younger than those who die young, after having begotten children. The person who is advanced in age but has no children, lives only one life, and his death marks the end of his life. But, those who would have begotten children have the capacity to live forever.

For a person to qualify as an ancestor, he should have lived an exemplary life that is worth of emulation.[3] This requirement is one of the least important in the making of an ancestor because it is too subjective. There is no consensus among African people as to how an exemplary life should look. Hence, it becomes the prerogative of the offspring of the dead person to decide whether to initiate their dead relative into ancestorhood or not. However, most Africans have moral guidelines and standards that help them decide whether a person is good or bad, and right or wrong. The Shona talk of *unhu* that can be translated as good manners. *Unhu* is the essence of being a human being. It involves respect for self and others, particularly one's seniors.

According to Michael Gelfand, *unhu* is connected to ancestors and the lack of it offends ancestors who are next to God.[4] People with *unhu* are not involved in immoral activities, and if they do, they repent and take full responsibility for their actions. They avoid stealing, incest, ill-treating their parents, killing other human beings intentionally or accidentally, and if they do, they accept accountability for their actions. People with *unhu* are not verbally and physically violent. They are responsible people who work hard to provide for their families and communities. They pay their bridewealth if they are married men. If the dead person's family thinks that one does not qualify to become an ancestor because of the lack of *unhu*, then, they may refrain from performing the cleansing ritual. If the spirit of that person tries to bulldoze its way to ancestorhood by compelling its living relatives to perform the ceremony, they have an option to exorcize it.

Among the Shona, if the deceased is a known murderer, who has not paid compensation to appease the spirit of the dead person, his relatives are not likely to be eager to bring his spirit back home as an ancestor. Some people fear that if they allow such a spirit to come back into the home as

---

3. Opoku, *West African Traditional Religion*, 36.
4. Gelfand, "UNHU—The Personality of the Shona."

an ancestor, he will be accompanied by the avenging spirit of the murdered person, and that would have devastating consequences to the members of the family. Although some traditional healers claim to have the powers to separate the ancestor from the avenging spirit, that exorcism is not always successful. The relatives may also refuse to perform the cleansing ceremony for notorious witches due to the fear that such spirits may pass on the witchcraft to one of the family members. However, witchcraft is practiced secretly, and in most cases, those people who are accused of practicing it deny the charge, and may have the sympathy of their relatives. Furthermore, in most situations, a person can be a witch without his family knowing about it, and in that case, the cleansing ceremony will be performed. It is hard to know if one's deceased parent was a witch or not. In the end, even people who are believed to be witches by outsiders, can be allowed to become ancestors by their families.

To qualify for ancestorhood, one should die a normal death. Normal death refers to death that is not caused by any one of the tabooed causes. Among the Shona, if one dies from tuberculosis, epilepsy, and leprosy, he cannot become an ancestor.[5] The Shona think that if such a person becomes an ancestor, he might bring the disease that killed him into the family, and may pass it on to another family member. The Shona do not concur on whether those people who commit suicide can become ancestors or not. Some families allow such people to become ancestors, and others do not. Those who allow such people to become ancestors argue that the deceased was not responsible for his death, for the death would have been caused by evil spirits. They believe that no one can take his own life unless he is blinded and confused by evil or avenging spirits. Prior to the performance of the cleansing ceremony for such a spirit, some families perform a ritual to separate the spirit of their relative from the evil spirits that might have caused his death. Those Shona ethnic groups, which argue against initiating into ancestorhood a person who would have died of suicide fear that such a spirit might cause another family member to commit suicide. In West Africa, those who die of suicide, accidents, violence, lunacy, dropsy, leprosy, and epilepsy are prevented from becoming ancestors.[6]

Ancestral Rituals

For one to become an ancestor it is crucial that his corpse be accorded proper burial rituals, which should be performed meticulously by authorized

---

5. Ikenga-Metuh, *Comparative Studies of African Traditional Religions*, 147.
6. Opoku, *West African Traditional Religion*, 36.

sacred practitioners. The rituals begin immediately as soon as one dies. The dead person's eyes and mouth should be closed, and his hands are folded before the body becomes rigid. Consequently, the dying person should be watched constantly so that those who have the authority to do so may perform the rituals. Before burial, some African groups wash the corpse, smear it with body oil, and dress it appropriately. The corpse is never left alone until burial. The marking of the grave (*kutema ruhahu*) is one of the most crucial rituals among the Shona. One of the designated elders of the deceased person identifies and marks the place where the grave should be dug. As the designated sacred practitioner marks the place where the grave should be dug, he utters, "This is where we are going to bury you. This is your new home." After that ritual, anyone can take part in the digging of the grave. If the dead person is a woman, only members of her family of origin are authorized to identify and mark the grave site. Her husband or children are not allowed to do that since she is not related to them by blood.

If a person dies away from home, in a place where he lives among strangers, anyone who has the same totem, or comes from the same country may perform the *ruhahu* ritual. Once the body is placed into the grave, it may face the direction that the elders of the family prescribe. Some Shona ethnic groups may place some of the items or clothes belonging to the dead person into the grave. The Karanga of Nyajena tear apart all the items before placing them into the grave. They also make holes through the plates that are put into the grave. Some Shona groups have people who watch over the grave on the first night just to prevent witches from desecrating the buried body. The Karanga sweep the area around the grave and sprinkle it with the water that the grave diggers would have used to wash their hands after the burial. Early in the morning, some of the relatives go to the grave to check if anyone would have stepped closer to the grave. On the next day of burial or a couple of weeks or months after the burial, the estate of the deceased is distributed after sprinkling it with herbs (*kubata nhumbi*). It is believed that the unsanctioned use of a dead person's clothes may cause misfortunes to the persons involved.

If the dead person has never fathered any children, a rat is placed into his anus or just beside him in the grave. If the dead person is a woman who would have died without begetting children, the same ritual is performed. Alternatively, they may bury a log that is used to pound grain (*mutswi*) alongside the body. During the ritual, the following words may be said: "Son, you have died, and you have left no child or wife. Here is your wife and child. Go away for good. Please, never come back because there is nothing to come back for. No one needs your protection." This ritual reminds the spirit of the dead that without having begotten children, he is not allowed to become an ancestor.

Although the omission of some burial rituals may not prevent the dead from becoming an ancestor, it angers his spirit and delays the process of becoming an ancestor. A big challenge is presented by those people who just disappear, and whose death has not been confirmed. Their relatives delay performing the burial rituals for them because they still have the hope that one day they will come back home alive. However, when all the hope is gone, people may perform some of the burial rituals, and allow the dead to become an ancestor if he qualifies. Usually, they consult a traditional medical practitioner to determine whether the disappeared person is dead or not.

Among the Shona, the most crucial requirement for becoming an ancestor is the performance of the cleansing ceremony that has been alluded to above. The cleansing ceremony is a ritual that is performed at least six months after the burial of a dead person, which transforms his spirit into an ancestor. It is popularly known as *kugadzira* or *kurova guva*. *Kugadzira* literally means to make. In this case, it refers to the making of the ancestor. *Kurova guva* is made up of *kurova*, which means to beat up, and *guva*, which means grave. It refers to the rituals that take place at the grave on the day the ancestor is brought home. *Kurova guva* is performed for both men and women. The Shona believe that about six months after someone's death and burial, the body is likely to have fully decomposed. It is important that the body is completely decomposed at the time of the *kurova guva* because the people fear that if the ritual is performed before the decomposition of the buried body, the ancestor might come into the home with his body. If that happens, it would be difficult to distinguish the ancestor from another spirit that is called *dhupwa* (ghost), which is believed to have a human body. An ancestor with a physical body is not desirable because it may scare the living family members.

There is much preparation before the ritual is performed. Once the responsible family members realize that the ceremony is due, they begin to make the necessary preparations. For a woman, it is the responsibility of her male children, in consultation with her relatives, to perform the ceremony. The children would provide the required beast, food, and beer, and the mother's relatives would preside over the ritual. If the deceased is a man, his children are responsible for providing the required things. The family ritual practitioner normally presides over the performance of ritual.

The members of the extended family are required to contribute a portion of grains (*rapoko*) that are used to brew the ritual beer. They may brew the beer in their respective homes, and then bring a few clay containers (*pfuko*) filled with beer to the home where the ritual is performed. About two days before the ritual, a few close family members of the dead person may go to consult a traditional healer, if that ritual would not have been performed a few days after the burial. The purpose of that consultation is to find out if the spirit of the deceased is tainted with some evil spirits, or angry because of the lack of meticulous burial rituals. If the spirit is tainted, then the traditional healer may recommend the performance of a ritual to separate the ancestral spirit from the evil spirits. Again, if the spirit is angry because of one reason or another, the responsible family members should appease it by paying compensation (*kubata makuku*). Some families might also inquire about the cause of the death at this point, if it was not carried out a few days after the burial.

The cleansing ceremony is attended by most family members and the local villagers. The family members start to gather a couple of days before the ceremony. On the day of the ceremony, a group of close family members together with the sacred practitioner goes to the grave at dawn with a small clay pot (*pfuko*) of beer. Once they arrive there, they sing and dance around the grave. They pour some beer unto the grave, and tell the deceased that they have come to take him home. Amid much pomp and fanfare, the delegation then pulls a branch of a tree on which it is believed that the ancestor is riding. Once they arrive home where the cleansing ceremony is being performed, everybody joins them in welcoming the ancestor.

If the relatives of the ancestor suspect or have been advised that the ancestor might be angry, the goat of anger (*mbudzi yeshungu/svitsa*) should be sacrificed. The live goat is brought to the threshold of the traditional kitchen in which most of the rituals take place. The male eldest grandchild or nephew of the deceased holds the goat by the front leg, while all family members, stand in a single file, and in turns, pour beer on its back, starting with the most senior. Those members of the family who are not present can be represented by any of the relatives who are present in the pouring of beer. It is believed that if the ancestor has decided to reconcile with the family, then the goat should vigorously shake its body as a sign of its acceptance of the ceremony. Usually, the goat shakes its body in response to the pouring of beer on its back. Once it does that everyone goes ecstatic. The ancestor has forgiven his family, and has accepted the cleansing ceremony. If the goat refuses to shake its body, although it is rare, it is a sign that the ancestor is not happy, and has rejected the ritual. In that case, the family would have to perform another ritual in the future. Since the shaking of the goat is crucial, it becomes imperative that even those members of the family who are not present at the ceremony should have someone representing them during the ritual. Once the goat shakes its body, as it almost always does, and the ancestor is deemed happy, then the goat is slaughtered. Its meat is *braaied* or barbecued (*kugocha*) and eaten without salt.

The next ritual is the slaughtering of the sacrificial beast. Some Shona groups pour beer on the back of the beast as they do to the goat, and others do not. Usually, if the ancestor has already accepted the ritual through the *shungu* goat, then it might not be necessary to repeat the same ritual. But if there is no *shungu* goat, then the beast should be subjected to the process, which has been described above. Once the cow is slaughtered, some special pieces of meat are cut from the heart, liver, kidneys, and the plate of the cow, and are cooked separately. When the sacred meat is ready to eat, the sacred practitioner distributes the pieces of meat accompanied with a morsel of sacred *sadza* (think porridge prepared from rapoko) to the close family members. This meal is the Holy Communion, which reunites both the invisible and visible members of the family. After that meal, other guests may consume the rest of the saltless meat. The rest of the day is spent dancing and singing, celebrating the transformation of the dead into an ancestor.

The name inheritance ritual happens the day after the *kurova guva* ceremony. The name of the ancestor is given to one of the family members. If the ancestor is a woman, her name is given to her eldest granddaughter, who might have been given the same name at her birth. For a male ancestor, the name is inherited by his eldest son, even if the father's name is already being used by one of the sons or cousins. In some cases, the *rukanda* (bangle made from the leg skin of the sacrificed beast) that the eldest nephew of the deceased would have made is given to the eldest son of the ancestor. Ordinarily, the nephew is paid a cow for that job. At this moment, the people may celebrate the inheritance of the name by offering gifts such as money and other items to the inheritor, amid much dancing, singing, and beer drinking. The named inheritor, with the blessings of the ancestor, becomes the new head of the family.

For widows, there is *kudarika vuta* (jumping over the weapons) ceremony that should be performed at about this point. One of the tools or weapons that belong to the deceased, for example, an axe, spear, bow, or arrow is placed across the doorway of the ritual house. The widow is asked to jump over the weapon to and from the sacred house. It is believed that if the woman has been unfaithful to her dead husband during the period between his death and the cleansing ritual, any attempt to jump over the weapon would cause her to fall or break her backbone. The refusal to perform the ritual is likely to be interpreted as the confirmation that the widow would have been unfaithful to her late husband. That refusal brings much scorn and shame upon the woman, her children, and relatives. It should be noted that the ritual of *kudarika vuta* is not performed for men, which has led some feminist activists and theologians to allege that it is biased against women.

The final ritual that is connected to the cleansing ceremony is the inheritance of the widow by any authorized relative of the late husband. Those who qualify are the late husband's brothers, cousins, the eldest son, and nephews. In the past, there were instances where one of the eldest son from the most senior wife of the deceased would be asked to inherit one of his late father's youngest wives. The authorized members of the family sit in a circle, with the widow kneeling in the middle of that circle. She holds a dish of warm water and a hand towel in her hands. She hands over the water to the person that she wants to become her husband, and after he has washed his hands, she wipes them with the towel. The chosen man is not supposed to reject the widow because she still belongs to his late relative, and he only becomes her new provider, protector, and guardian. It should be noted that the widow may decide to choose her eldest son to become her guardian. By walking that path, she communicates that she is no longer interested in a sexual relationship, but just wants her son to become her guardian. Once she does that, then she should remain chaste as long as she lives in the home of her deceased husband. However, it has become difficult to monitor the widow's sexual life since relatives no longer live in the same locality. If she chooses any one of the brothers or nephews of her late husband, that man becomes her husband. She may remain in her late husband's home, and the inheritor who may have his own family at this point, would shuttle between the two homes.

The cleansing ceremony marks the beginning of the deceased's ancestorhood. Once one becomes an ancestor, she continues to be one until the last member of his family who remembers him dies. The death of such a family member marks the transformation and degeneration of the ancestor into a nameless spirit, which has no influence on any family. Offspring is crucial if the remembrance of the ancestor is to be prolonged. The bigger the family of the deceased, the longer the remembrance. It should be noted that the cleansing ceremony is crucial in the process of becoming an ancestor. The living family members are critical stakeholders in that process, for it is their prerogative to initiate one as an ancestor, or to refuse to do that. Male children are crucial in the performance of the *kurova guva* ceremony, although female children, with the assistance of their paternal uncles, may also perform the ritual.

The Abode of Ancestors

The most prominent dwelling place of the ancestors is the home of their family members. Once the cleansing ceremony is performed, the Shona believe that the ancestors come to live in the homes of their family members. Since they are spiritual, they have no specific house or room that is allocated to them. However, the round and grass-thatched kitchen hut is believed to be the ancestors' favorite house. Most ancestral rituals are performed in or at the threshold of the kitchen hut. At this point, ancestors are no longer limited by space or time. They can get into and out of every room even when its doors are locked. Wherever their living family members are eating, sitting, working, walking, and sleeping, their ancestors are with them. They can be in all their relatives' homes, at the same time. They do not have to walk to arrive at a place, but they just wish to be there, and they are there. Since they are always present in the home, they know what their visible relatives lack and need, and how they feel. They know their secrets.

Sometimes families dedicate a bull (*kunzi*) to an ancestor, and that animal acquires the name of the ancestor. The bull is treated with respect because it hosts the family ancestor. It is exempted from hard labor such as ploughing or pulling the Scotch cart. It is given the privilege of bringing fertility to the family cows. Such bulls have double identities. First, they are animals because they still behave like other animals and live in the cattle kraal. Second, they are humans, for they are rendered the respect that is reserved for ancestors. They are called by the ancestor's name and title. So, ancestors can be thought of as living on those host bulls that live in the kraal. When the relatives want to get rid of the ancestor bull, they carry out a ritual in which they remove the ancestor from the bull before they slaughter it. Its meat is eaten without salt, and some of it is distributed to all family members.

Ancestors are sometimes referred to as *vari kumhepo* (those in the air), and that makes them ubiquitous. They reside in the sky and ride on the wind. From that vantage point, they can watch over every family member wherever they are. No one escapes their scrutiny. They travel as fast as the wind. They are life-giving as the air that people breathe. This vantage dwelling place enables them to know their relatives' secrets. The family members who live in accordance with the traditional moral standards of the elders are blessed by the ancestors. Transgressors of those moral standards cannot escape the microscopic scrutiny of the ancestors.

Ancestors also live underneath the earth since they were buried in the soil. First, it was their umbilical codes that were buried in the soil and later, their bodies. The soil is the dwelling place that connects them with every other ancestors and members of their families whose umbilical codes were buried in the same soil. The Shona refer to ancestors as *vari muvhu* (those in the soil), or just *ivhu,* which means soil. Although they reside in the soil, they are not limited by it. In fact, they own the soil and contribute to its fertility. They make the soil fruitful by bringing the rain. When the Shona give offerings to the ancestors, they pour or place them on the ground. The blood of sacrificial animals, and the beer are poured onto the ground. Ground tobacco (*fodya yebute*), which is a delicacy for ancestors, is also placed on the ground.

Among the Shona, some mountains and hills are sacred because the ancestors reside on them. First, some of the ancestors were buried in the caves on those hills, which transformed them into sacred places. Second, the Shona believe that the higher one goes, the holier it becomes. Since ancestors live in the sky, it then logically follows that any object that is higher or taller may attract them as an abode. People who climb up those mountains should observe the code of conduct that is explained to them by their guides or elders. In the past, one of those codes of conduct involved being respectful to the surrounding nature by refraining from cursing and picking up the fruits without following the prescribed rules. Those who failed to follow these codes of conduct could be punished by the ancestors by losing their way (*kubatwa nechidzimira*). Sometimes transgressors would be harassed by wild animals as the punishment for their disrespectful behavior. The Karanga of Nyajena have Chitakai Mountain, which attracts sacred edible insects called *harugwa* that are believed to come from God through the ancestors. Every year, around the month of May, *harugwa* are seen in the sky orbiting the sun, before they land on the trees of Chitakai Mountain. Before the people can harvest the delicious sacred insects, a thanksgiving ritual to the ancestors (*kushuma*) is performed by the authorized sacred practitioner. It is believed that any attempt to harvest the insects before the *kushuma* ritual upsets the ancestors, who may withdraw the insects.

Ancestors are also associated with rivers and pools. One of the most popular rivers from which the national ancestors (*mhondoro*) are said to quench their thirst is the gigantic Zambezi River, and because of that, it is sacred. Ancestors also drink from pools that are scattered all over the country. People should respect those sacred pools by observing certain regulations. For instance, they should not use dirty containers to fetch water from such pools. No soap should be used in those pools because it irritates the spirits.

An ancestor can choose any of the family members as a host. The person becomes sick and the family consults a traditional healer who advises them that the sick person has been chosen by the ancestor as a host. Beer is brewed and the ancestor openly possesses the chosen person. Male ancestors can choose either male or female hosts, but female ancestors can only choose female hosts. Whenever the family would like to communicate with the ancestor, they ask the host to summon the ancestor. This invitation is usually done by placing ground tobacco (*fodya yebute*) on the shoulders of the host who immediately becomes possessed. Some hosts may invite the ancestor by wearing the ancestral regalia, and humming a sacred tune. The ancestor may also possess the host at any time that it deems necessary. The hosts have taboos that they should observe. They avoid eating certain types of food such as millet products. They also do not eat an improperly slaughtered goat. The Shona respect such ancestral hosts because they are sacred practitioners. Although some places can be pinpointed as ancestral dwelling places, since ancestors are spirits, they live everywhere.[7]

The Role of Ancestors

The Shona worldview is replete with all sorts of spirits—some good and others malevolent. The African's life is an unending marathon, fleeing the onslaught from the evil spirits, while soliciting the assistance of benevolent spirits. Ancestors are the champions of those invisible protectors in whom the living find refuge from the onslaught of the bad spirits. Ancestors have a leg in the world of the living and another in the land of the spirits, and consequently, they understand how both worlds work. They see what ordinary human beings cannot see. They see the whole: past, present, and future, and because of that they protect their living family members from impending misfortunes. Ancestors do not prevent misfortunes from happening, but they enable their family members to escape them unharmed. They control the movement of their relatives, and make sure that they do not go where there is harm.

It is one of the roles of the ancestors to monitor and enforce morality. Every human society has moral standards that should be adhered to unwaveringly. Among the Shona people, taking another person's life intentionally or accidentally is prohibited, and is punishable because life is sacred. Neglecting one's social responsibilities is another blameworthy offense. Adultery is strongly loathed by the society and ancestors. Shona communities have traditional leaders, and one of their duties is to enforce the traditional moral standards. Most people follow those moral codes of conduct, but a few people sometimes disregard them. Although some offenders can escape apprehension and punishment by the traditional law enforcement agents

---

7. Opoku, *West African Traditional Religion*, 36.

because no one would have seen them when they commit the offenses, they cannot escape the penetrating and unfailing gaze of the ancestors. J. O. Kayode emphasizes the same point saying, "Ancestors punish the neglectful and disobedient and are particularly severe on breaches of discipline and of duties which each member of the family owes to one another."[8] Those people who secretly transgress the moral standards of the land would be punished by the ancestors. This role of ancestors was more crucial in the traditional society where there were no full-time law enforcement agents. It is the duty of ancestors to warn perpetrators before they commit criminal offenses, apprehend those who disregard their warning, and mete out appropriate punishment.

The land belongs to ancestors because it was given to them by our creator. No human being created the soil, and all that naturally grows on it. The traditional Shona believed that no individual had absolute ownership rights to the land because it belonged to the ancestors. No one should be deprived of taking advantage of its nourishment for the survival of one's family. Ancestors, who are the custodians of the land, have the duty to fertilize and make it fruitful. It is their responsibility to protect what grows on it from diseases and drought. Ancestors bring the rain that makes it fecund. They make fruit trees produce fruits for the nourishment and sustenance of human beings. Everything that grows on the land should be respected and used responsibly to nourish humanity. The ancestors understand the needs of the soil because that is their dwelling place. Everyone should find a place where she can build a home and grow crops. Among the Shona, although in towns all land is for sale, land is free in the rural areas. Anyone who would like to use it may approach any local traditional leaders and ask for land, and if it is available he will be allocated a piece of land on which to build a house and practice farming.

The human family needs to perpetuate itself by engaging in an ongoing reproduction of offspring. Unless human beings continue to bring forth children into the world, there will not be anyone to use the land. Consequently, human fertility is a crucial responsibility of the ancestors among the Shona. Every marriage should be fruitful, and ancestors see to it that children are born in each family. They direct those who want to marry to the places where they can find partners. They are interested in the process of marriage, especially the payment of bridewealth. They are present when married couples engage in sexual activities. The Shona have poems and prayers *(zvirevereve zvepabonde)* that they sometimes recite during intercourse to acknowledge the presence of the ancestors. Ancestors are

---

8. Kayode, *Understanding African Traditional Religion*, 19.

present when babies are being formed in the deep of the womb, and they protect the pregnant mother from the harm that can be caused by the invisible, anti-human forces. At birth, they welcome the newly born baby into the union of the family members, through the burial of the umbilical code, and protect her from all harm. The Shona believe that babies are so close to the ancestors to the extent that they may sense the presence of immoral people and evil forces.

Some ancestors are endowed with the knowledge of herbs that heal. Some of them lived at a time when there were no modern medicines and had to learn how to use herbs to cure their ailments. These herbs worked for them, and that is why when the Europeans came to Zimbabwe, the indigenous people were thriving. Unfortunately, the Shona never thought of establishing a method of writing, so that they could preserve their knowledge of the helpful herbs. Some of that knowledge was orally passed on from generation to generation, and consequently, most of the knowledge was lost. It is only ancestors that can reach back to primordial times and retrieve some of that information. They then bring it back through the inspiration or dreams of some family members. In addition to that, ancestors fight the baleful spirits that cause a lot of harm among human beings.

In a society that relied on nature for its livelihood, it was the duty of the ancestors to bless and lead the hunters and gatherers to the places where animals and fruits could be found. Since they are the owners of the forests, they knew where game and fruits could be found. The hunters performed rituals so that the ancestors could direct them where game was. They had to observe certain moral and hunting guidelines to avoid offending the ancestors. When they finally located the game, and slaughtered it, ancestors always had their share in the blood that was shed onto the soil. There were ancestral birds that could lead hunters to where game and honey could be found. Whenever the hunters located the game, it was not their intention to kill all, because they knew that they would want to come back the next day and still find animals. Since all the animals belonged to the ancestors, all the people could hunt them to feed their families. No private ownership of wild animals was recognized.

There were also guidelines for gathering wild fruits. First, no individual claimed the ownership of the jungles in which fruit trees were located. The trees belonged to the ancestors. The selling of wild fruits was forbidden. The Shona were disillusioned when the Europeans came to Zimbabwe, and parceled out land to themselves as private property. As if that was not greedy enough, they claimed to have ownership of the animals and fruits that they found in those farms. The Shona could not understand how an individual could claim to privately own the fish of the waters and animals of the jungle, which were given by the ancestors and God for the nourishment of everyone. In hunting and gathering, ancestors played another significant role of giving protection to the hunters and gathers from being attacked by dangerous wild animals such as snakes, hyenas, and lions. Even today, it is believed that ancestors guide their family members to where jobs are found. They inspire students and workers to achieve their utmost best, and protect them from all industrial hazards.

Ancestors have a hierarchy. At the bottom of the hierarchical ladder are those recent dead family members that have been initiated into ancestorhood. These ancestors are the most well-known to their living relatives because some of them would have died recently. Above the immediate ancestors, there are those ancestors that the living members of the family know partially. At the top of the hierarchy are those ancestors that most family members no longer remember by their names. It becomes the duty of the most well-known ancestors to intercede for their relatives before senior ancestors and God. At the end of the Shona prayer to the ancestors, the sacred practitioner asks the known ancestors to pass the message to those that the living family members can no longer remember. The rainmaking ceremony is principally intended to ask the ancestors to intercede for the people so that *Mwari* (God) may grant them rain. However, in most family traditional rituals, *Mwari* is not mentioned because the issues at stake lie within the jurisdiction of the ancestors.

Communication with the Ancestors

Ancestors do communicate with the living members of their families whenever there is a need. One way of ancestral communication is through dreams. In some of these dreams people interact with the ancestors as one would do with a living person. Most Shona people believe that one does not dream of the deceased members of one's family unless ancestors are communicating something. Other dreams concern animals that can be interpreted as symbols of ancestors.

In cases where the family elders cannot interpret the dreams, people may seek the help of traditional medical practitioners. Usually, each community has ritual practitioners that can be relied on for the accurate interpretation of dreams.

Sometimes ancestors communicate through its host. The host gets into a trance and begins to act weirdly. This possession may happen during ancestral rituals or any other time deemed necessary by the ancestor and the family. Once possessed, the host of the ancestral spirit may begin to imitate the mannerism of the ancestor during his bodily life, such as voice, dance, eating habits, favorite food, among other things. Members of the family may then ask the spirit some questions pertaining to the welfare of family members, and the possible challenges that members might encounter in the future.

At times, ancestors communicate through calamity. Usually, this happens when ancestors are upset about something that one of the members of the family would have committed, such as murder, incest, ill-treatment of the elderly, and adultery. The calamity may be in the form of disease, pestilence, death, drought, bad luck, or accident. When the Shona experience inexplicable misfortunes, they consult traditional sacred practitioners, who may alert them of the need to appease the aggrieved ancestors. Ancestors can also be conducted by their family members through the pouring of libation, ground tobacco, and animal blood onto the ground. The Shona perform such rituals at the threshold of the round hut kitchen, which is their sacred place. The sacred practitioner may say words of prayer during such an offering while other family members are kneeling and quiet. At the end of the prayer, everyone may clap hands, whistle, and ululate. This method of communication is like a one-way traffic because there is no immediate response from the ancestors.

Relationship between Ancestors and the Living

The relationship between ancestors and their physical relatives is that of respect, love, and fear. Ancestors are respected because they are senior members of the family, and they do have mysterious power, which is derived from their dual affiliation to the physical and spiritual realms. They understand and speak the languages of both worlds. They are feared because they see what the physical people do not see, and do have the authority and power to punish the transgressors of societal norms. "They punish the neglectful and disobedient and are particularly severe on breaches of discipline and of the duties which each member of the family owes to one another and their head."[9] They perform a dual duty—they apprehend transgressors of traditional standards, and at the same time mete out appropriate punishments. They play the police officer and judge at the same time.

Many things can anger the ancestors. They are upset if the beast of motherhood is not paid by the son-in-law or if it is disposed of inappropriately. The beast of motherhood (*mombe youmai*) is the only bridewealth cow that the mother of the bride gets from the son-in-law, and its purpose is to

9. Kayode, *Understanding African Traditional Religion*, 19.

appease the maternal ancestors of the bride.[10] Ancestors also feel aggravated if the living family members refuse to perform the *kurova guva* ceremony, a ritual which initiates the newly deceased of the family into ancestorhood. Other things such as the failure to give the dead proper burial rites, and incest, refusal to take *chimutsamapfiwa*, adultery, neglect of parents in times of their need, failure to observe the sacred day, and the spilling of innocent blood may make ancestors angry.

According to Michael Gelfand, ancestors are also "opposed to a man's leaving his birthplace or *nyika* as he tends to break the lineage and so the unity and strength of the clan."[11] Leaving home would also be interpreted as forsaking the land in which one's umbilical code is buried. Among the Shona, the burying of the umbilical code is a symbolic act that signifies the unity between the newly born baby, the people belonging to that family clan, and the ancestors. The ground is sacred and acts as a communication center between the ancestors and their bodily relatives. If a Shona person, who lives away from home encounters misfortunes, he is advised to visit his rural home, or the place where his umbilical code is buried. It is believed that the visit can turn around his fortunes. It should be noted that the industrialization and urbanization of the Shona society made it possible for young people to leave their rural homes. However, wherever they go, they should always support their relatives back home, and occasionally visit them. Ancestors too should be notified of any planned trip, and solicit their protection and blessings for the traveler.

Ancestors can be greatly offended if a person beats up or ill-treats his parent or grandparents. Elders should be respected since by virtue of their age, they are closer to the ancestral realm. Their closeness to the ancestors compel the ancestors to answer their prayers favorably. If they become angry because of some ill-treatment that is caused by one of their offspring, the ancestors take it upon themselves to punish the culprit. Although respect should be awarded all the elders of the clan, it is only the ill-treatment of one's parents that attracts the wrath of the ancestors. If the ill-treated parent is one's mother, her spirit may come back to haunt the transgressor after her death. Although the spirit of an ill-treated father does not become an avenging spirit to his children, he relies for justice on the timely intervention of the ancestors.

The nature and quality of the relationship between the living and the living dead depends on the moral disposition of the concerned people. Those who are morally upright have no reason to fear the ancestors because

---

10. Gelfand, "UNHU—The Personality of the Shona."
11. Ibid.

they do not punish morally upright people. In most cases, it is the violators of traditional moral standards who fear the ancestors. However, there are times when ancestors punish the whole family or clan because of the transgression of one person, and because of that reason, everyone is everyone's keeper. Every family member has an ancestral-given mandate to reprimand the wayward members of the family. In situations where ancestors should be appeased for a wrong that has been committed by one member of the community, which affects the whole family or clan, all affected members should contribute resources for the appeasement of the offended spirits. One good thing about the ancestors is that they are always ready to forgive if the transgressor repents by offering a sacrifice to appease them.[12]

The Encounter with Christianity

One of the Shona ritual practices that the early Christian missionaries condemned was the veneration of ancestors. For most of them, it was not veneration, but worship of ancestors. Their religion informed them that God was Trinitarian—God the Father, God the Son, and God the Holy Spirit. All worship was supposed to be directed to God, not to idols or dead human beings. Ancestors were condemned as evil, and having no ability to intercede for the people. For missionaries, there was only one way to the Father—Jesus Christ. Ancestral rituals were demonized and, in some cases, the missionaries established Christian villages in which believers were placed so that they would not have bad influences from the non-believers, who lived outsides the walls of the sacred villages.

The response by the Shona was multi-faceted. Some thought that the veneration of ancestors was not different from the Christian churches' practice of honoring the saints. The missionaries taught that the saints were the triumphant members of the Christian church, and could intercede for the living members of the church before God. They ignored the fact that the ancestors performed the *same* responsibility. Consequently, some Shona people thought that the missionaries were hypocrites who, on the one hand, condemned the ancestral veneration, and on the other, enforced the veneration of Christian saints. Many people felt that the missionaries were insincere to think that God could not create saints or ancestors from the Shona before their arrival. To worsen the matter, the Christian saints were not related to the people for whom they were supposed to intercede.

Some Shona people led two lives, which were influenced by two different religious traditions. They faked the rejection of the traditional ways of

12. Ibid.

life publicly, yet steadfastly and secretly observing them. They continued to perform the rites of passage, particularly concerning marriage and death, that ensured the deceased a place in the ancestral realm. In times of desperation, even those members of the family who had professed undivided commitment to the new faith reverted to their traditional ways. Sometimes, the traditional rituals are concurrently performed with the Christian rituals. At some rituals, such as weddings and burials, syncretic tendencies are apparent. For instance, at burials, the Shona perform rituals from both the traditional religion and Christianity. This attitude has forced some Shona Christians to be Christians during the day, and traditionalists by the night.

The other way the Shona people responded to the condemnation of their ancestral veneration was to rebel against the missionaries by founding their own Christian churches that are popularly known as African Independent Churches. Most of these churches intermarried their traditional and Christian religious beliefs to meet the needs of both the founder and followers. These churches will be discussed in detail in chapter 9. Consequently, some Christian churches allow polygamy, and exorcize their followers from the effects of witchcraft. They perform faith healing and prophecy. Some mainline churches, such as the Roman Catholic Church, have responded by embarking on a controversial theological program that is known as inculturation, localization, indigenization, or contextualization. The term means the encounter between the gospel of Jesus Christ and a culture, in which the gospel challenges, purifies, and adopts some cultural practices for the purpose of transforming the faith of the people. Although ancestor veneration is not as widespread as it was before the arrival of Christianity, it has remained powerful in rural areas. What is intriguing to Christian ministers is that most Shona Christians require their relatives to perform the cleansing ceremony after their death. Most people want both traditional and Christian rituals to be performed at their funerals. The question that continues to boggle the minds of African theologians is whether a spirit can be an ancestor, and be in heaven at the same time. It seems that Shona Christians think that it is possible. If ancestors were in hell, they would not be able to come back to their living families. It seems that in the area of ancestor veneration, most Christian churches have decided to remain indifferent.

5

Avenging Spirits

The Shona believe that the life of a human being is so sacred that it must not be voluntarily, legally, or accidentally taken away by anybody. They unfalteringly uphold every person's right to live because they believe in the intrinsic goodness and sacredness of every person's life. Although the modern laws of Zimbabwe allow the courts to sentence some criminals to death, the traditional Shona do not agree with them. That is why at some point after Zimbabwe gained its independence from Britain, the courts had a hard time trying to find a Shona person who was willing to work as a hangman. You cannot get paid for killing people, even if they are criminals, because their life is sacred too. They might have committed egregious crimes but their lives remain sacred and may not be taken from them without adverse consequences to the hangman and his family.

The belief in the sacredness of every human life and the taboo against taking it explain why some early writers of the history of Zimbabwe mistook the Shona's respect for human life and peacefulness for cowardice. That peacefulness made it easier for the Ndebele to resettle in Zimbabwe around 1840 without much harassment and rebellion from the Shona. A handful of Ndebele fighters would send a whole Shona village into the caves to hide, not because they were cowards, but because they were peaceful. I do not intend to portray the Ndebele as a people that did not respect human life, because they did, in their own way, per their own traditions. Rayner states that the Shona "rated civility and moderation above courage for instance, and do this to this day."[1] He goes on to describe the Shona as gentler and a people interested in relationships, who could have defeated the Ndebele if they had imitated their fighting styles; but "such a profound change was quite beyond them, alien to their make-up and no doubt distasteful to them."[2] But the Shona did not lack courage and fatal fighting strategies; rather, they valued life above everything else. The thought of having killed a human being, on purpose or by accident, is overwhelming for Shona people, and the fear of the spiritual repercussions may haunt them forever.

1. Rayner, *The Tribe and Its Successors*, 33–34.
2. Ibid., 34.

This fear explains why the British, who were so scared of even a handful of Ndebele fighters under King Lobengula, and avoided any route that would bring them closer to the Ndebele, could just march into Mashonaland without any slightest fear of the Shona. It is said that some of the early white settlers feared wild animals more than they feared the Shona. A quick look at the Ndebele-Shona Uprisings of 1896–98, further affirms the point made by Rayner. Although the white settlers knew for certain that the Ndebele would revolt after their unceremonious defeat during the Anglo-Ndebele War of 1893–94, they never suspected that the Shona would also revolt. They could not conceive of a situation that would provoke the Shona into taking up arms against anybody.

This belief in the sacredness of human life feeds into the belief in the avenging spirit, which they call *ngozi*. The Shona word *ngozi* literally means a horrendous accident. *Ngozi* is the spirit of a deceased person who was treated badly in life or was killed (intentionally or accidentally) and who now comes back to the perpetrator and his family, demanding justice and compensation for the wrong done or the loss incurred. The beliefs in *ngozi* and the sacredness of the human life complement each other. If you ill-treat someone, particularly your mother, then her spirit will haunt you after her death. If you kill someone, and no one apprehends you, justice will come from the spirit of the deceased person. In the traditional Shona society, there were no jails, but justice was still served. The Shona fear *ngozi* because: "An angry spirit is terrifying. Such a spirit attacks suddenly and very harshly. It usually attacks an individual through his family causing a succession of deaths, or death followed by serious illness in other members of the family. And the spirit is not easily appeased."[3] Of course, the traditional Shona engaged in wars, but their primary objective when fighting an enemy was not to massacre the opponents, but to scare them away. Killing them was avoided at all costs.

Types of *Ngozi*

Ngozi of One's Mother

Mothers are considered very important the world over, although they are sometimes neglected and ill-treated even by their own children. In the Shona society, mothers must be respected and cared for by their children during the years of their weakness and need that may be caused by old age or ill-health. In patrilineal Africa, most women leave their family homes

---

3. Bourdillon, *The Shona Peoples*, 233.

and relatives at marriage, to go and resettle with their husbands and their relatives. Most married women go to their husbands' homes as strangers. The longer they live in their new homes, the more relationships they establish. One of the strongest relationships that comes to them naturally is with their own children. Although married Shona women do not have the same totem with their children, they are their closest relatives in their new homes.[4] Women might be ill-treated by their husbands or his relatives, but their only consolation is in their own children. They expect support and empathy from their children, which at times are not forthcoming. For most Shona women, ill-treatment from one's own children is the worst betrayal one can conceive. Among the Shona, children should never ill-treat or neglect their mothers. If the children do offend their mothers, they should quickly ask for forgiveness and pay reparations. The failure to do so would prompt the spirit of the mother to come back as an avenging spirit after her death, demanding justice and compensation from the perpetrator.

There are many ways in which a Shona woman can be offended by one of her children. Insulting and beating up one's mother are totally abhorred and a disgrace, not only to the offender, but also to the whole community. Emotional and financial neglect of one's mother can cause the mother's spirit to become an avenging spirit. Some small things such as breaking her kitchen utensils—such as clay pots, porcelain cups, and plates—may lead to *kutanda botso*, which is a Shona penitentiary ritual for those who would have ill-treated their mothers. Traditionally, the kitchen utensils were precious to Shona women because they were among the few items that they could personally own in their marital homes. In the event of a divorce, the woman could take her kitchen utensils, the beast of motherhood and its offspring, her clothes, and her own wealth that might have come from the work of her hands, such as potting and knitting. All other properties would remain with the husband or his relatives. Any wanton or accidental destruction of such items and property would be punished by the mother's *ngozi*. Upon a mother's death, all the above-mentioned properties should be given to her own relatives, who may distribute some of them among the children of the deceased, and may retain the rest.

Failure to stand by one's mother when she is being ill-treated by one's father or other people can attract the wrath of her *ngozi* after her death. Although the Shona discourage their children from interfering during the domestic squabbles between their parents, any unwarranted abuse of the woman by her husband may attract the intervention of her older kids. Some

---

4. It has become common among the modern Shona for a man and a woman of the same totem to marry. In that case, then the children have the same totem with both parents.

abusive men are prevented by their older children from abusing their wives. Children should intervene to protect their mother, and failure to do so may be interpreted as betrayal and negligence by the mother, her relatives, and the community. Children should also protect their mother if she is persecuted by any one of the villagers. The issue that brings about most tensions in the Shona community involves the accusations of witchcraft. Children are expected to stand by their mother through thick and thin. She might be a witch to outsiders, but she remains a mother to her own children. The Shona have a proverb that says, "m*uroyi royera kure vomumba vagokugwira*," which can be literally translated as, "a witch should ply her bewitching business among people who are not members of her family so that her family members can defend her."

Refusing to pay the mother-in-law's beast of motherhood by the son-in-law may cause her spirit to come back as an avenging spirit, demanding compensation from her grandchildren. Shona men pay bridewealth for their wives as part of the marriage process, which might be in the form of cows, money, and any other items deemed appropriate by the woman's relatives. Of the head of cattle that the son-in-law is required to pay to the family of his bride, only one cow is given to the mother-in-law as an offering to maternal ancestors (*midzimu yokwamai*). This offering is intended to solicit the protection, guidance, and intercession of the children by the maternal ancestors. It is believed that when things get bad for any Shona person, the maternal ancestors stand by him, and will be the last to concede defeat. The beast of motherhood becomes the ancestors' property under the guardianship of the mother-in-law, and when she dies, that cow and its offspring should be passed on to her family of origin. If that cow is not paid, it frustrates the maternal ancestors, and causes the mother-in-law's spirit to come back after death asking for it.

Failure to take care of one's mother during her sickness may also cause the mother's spirit to come back as *ngozi*. Most rural Shona women do not have medical insurance and retirement savings. When they are sick, they expect their children and other relatives to assist them in paying medical bills. The Shona believe in the philosophy that obliges the parents to invest in their children by educating them, while expecting the family roles to switch at some point in time. As the parents become older, weaker, sicklier, and poorer, their children should take care of them. In addition to taking care of one's mother's medical expenses, children must also foot the funeral expenses of their parents, since most do not have any funeral insurance policies. All children should contribute towards the burial expenses, each according to his or her means. The refusal to either contribute or attend the funeral of one's mother offends her spirit, which is likely to come back to discipline the culprit as *ngozi*.

One good thing about the avenging spirit of the mother is that there are two ways in which it can be mollified. The more effective way to avoid the avenging spirit of one's mother is prevention, which requires all children to be a respectful, responsible, and accountable, particularly to their mother. If one is found wanting in one way or the other, the best thing to do is to ask for forgiveness, and to reconcile with one's mother before her death. If one breaks one of his mother's utensils, he should confess to his mother, and replace it if requested to. The reconciliation with one's mother is tinged with the payment of compensation. The forgiveness that the mother may readily dish out without being offered monetary or property compensation, does not stop the spirit of the mother from fighting for justice after death. The compensation could be in the form of a goat, cow, or money, and is called *kubata makuku*. This Shona phrase originally meant to give an offended person a chicken as compensation for any wrong done. Nowadays, the phrase refers to any item that might be given to anybody as reparations for a wrong done.

If reconciliation is not achieved before the death of the mother, or if compensation is not paid immediately after burial, then the embarrassing *kutanda botso* penitentiary ritual might be carried out by the culprit to conciliate the aggravated spirit of the mother. Literally *kutanda botso* can be translated as, to chase away violence. The perpetrator must brew some beer out of the grains that he collects from other people through begging. He is not allowed to use his own grains or money to cover the expenses of such a ritual. If he uses his own grains, then the ritual would be rendered invalid. He should dress in old rugs, sackcloth, or old strips of blanket, and walk from one home to another singing a beggar's song while asking for grains.[5] He has to let everyone know that he is a fool who had ill-treated his mother. The villagers are bound to give him something, but not before they ridicule him by throwing cold water or ashes on him.

Different kinds of grain are put in the same container, so that the perpetrator spends some time separating them. At the end of every begging day, he should carry back home on his shoulders, all the grains that he would have collected. Once the needed grains are gathered, the perpetrator, with the assistance of relatives, brews some beer to appease the spirit of the angry mother. On the day of the ritual, a goat or a cow may be given to the relatives of the deceased mother as a token of repentance. Some Shona groups demand that an ox belonging to the son in trouble, be slaughtered and then

---

5. Gelfand, *Shona Ritual with Special Reference to the Chaminuka Cult*, 153.

consumed by the people while drinking the beer.[6] The son who is performing the ritual should neither drink the appeasement beer nor eat the sacrificial meat. This ritual is more about shaming the unrepentant son, than the payment of compensation. It also acts as a deterrent to would-be mother abusers. The best way to avoid performing *kutanda botso* is respecting one's mother, and take care of her in times of her weakness and need.

Ngozi of a Vagabond and Alien

The avenging spirit of a vagabond (*rombe*) is devastating and very difficult to resolve. A *rombe* is usually a homeless person who has refused to take personal, familial, and communal responsibilities. Most of them are not married, though they are far past the marrying stage. For most Africans, refusal to marry is not only disdainful to one's family and the community in which one lives, but is also contemptuous to the ancestors. It is only the incorrigible societal deviants, and physically impaired people who may resist marriage, starting a family, and building a home. Among the Shona, homelessness is believed to be a sign of carelessness because there is always a place in which one can build a home. There is a general understanding among the Shona that some vagabonds are under the influence of antisocial spirits, which are evident in their rejection of the assistance in settling and starting families. Some of the vagabonds are bitter and angry because they are aware that the society despises them. The society expects them to build a home, and then start a family. In the rural areas of Zimbabwe, land can be acquired from the village head for free.

If such a vagabond is ill-treated, his spirit may come back with a vengeance seeking justice. The avenging spirit of a vagabond is believed to be disastrous because of the evil spirits that might have possession of him before his death. Such spirits may combine efforts with the spirit of the offended vagabond, and may become very powerful and dangerous. It is also believed that the bitterness of the vagabond, which is a result of his rough life, makes his *ngozi* very harsh and difficult to propitiate. The fact that some vagabonds have no known relatives makes it difficult for those who want to appease their spirits because no one comes forward to receive the compensation. So, every person, irrespective of his mental and social status, should be treated with respect and fairness, and failure to do that may be disastrous to the offender and his family after the mistreated person's death.

Connected to the vindictive *ngozi* of the vagabond is the avenging spirit of an alien. When diamonds and gold were discovered in South Africa

---

6. Ibid., 154.

in the nineteenth century, many people from Southern Africa travelled to South Africa to work in the mines. Most of them travelled by foot through Zimbabwe, which resulted in an influx of foreigners passing through the country. In addition to the movement of fortune seekers down South, the Federation of Rhodesia and Nyasaland (1953–63) attracted many people from both Malawi (Nyasaland) and Zambia (Northern Rhodesia) to Zimbabwe (Southern Rhodesia) to work in the mines and on the farms. The Shona called these economic immigrants *madeveranjanji*, which means people who travel on foot along the railway lines. Like any other sojourners, most of these people were vulnerable and relied on the generosity and protection of the Shona people through whose country they passed or came to resettle. Sometimes these immigrants needed food and protection from wild animals. Some of the immigrants would seek temporary employment among the Shona to replenish their food reserves as they looked for employment on the mines, or journeyed to South Africa. The lucky ones were employed to do menial work at some wealthy Shona families' homes and farms. However, some Shona people took advantage of the vulnerability of these immigrants and refused to remunerate them adequately as per agreement, for the work that they would have rendered. Some of these abused travelers later died, and their spirits came back to punish the abusive families. Efforts to pay compensation to pacify their *ngozi* were impeded by the unavailability of these spirits' relatives, who could receive the compensation. That is why the avenging spirit of the immigrant is believed to hit harder than most avenging spirits.

Any murdered person can become a *ngozi* spirit after his death. Whoever is responsible for the death of any person must pay compensation to the relatives of the deceased. It does not matter whether the person is intentionally or accidently killed, his life remains sacred, and the taboo against taking it should be upheld. People can be killed in a fight without the opponent's intention to kill them. Some people are run over by vehicles along the roads without any premeditation of the accident by the driver. There are several other accidents in which one may end up losing one's life. On the battlefield, a man must eliminate his opponents before they can kill him. The Shona believe that if the victims are combatants, there is a minimal chance of their spirits becoming *ngozi*, but there is no guarantee that they would not become *ngozi*. The soldiers who kill the unarmed and innocent civilians will one day bear the wrath of their avenging spirits. Wanton actions of cruelty perpetrated against the captured combatants and civilians during a war cannot go unpunished. Although the modern courts of Zimbabwe may exonerate a person who would have killed someone in an accident, the perpetrator should still pay compensation to the family of the deceased to abate the *ngozi*.

Ngozi of One's wife

The *ngozi* of an improperly buried wife is one of the most hazardous, and is among the most feared. When a married woman dies, her own people (brothers, sisters, or parents) must perform the ritual of marking her grave (*kutara ruhahu*). Her own children and husband are not authorized to perform that ritual to the satisfaction of the dead person because they are technically strangers to her. If the grave is not marked by the authorized relative of the deceased, her spirit may become a *ngozi* and would come back to haunt her husband's family including her own children. It has become fashionable in Zimbabwe that the wife's relatives refuse to perform the ritual if all bridewealth has not been paid by the son-in-law. In such cases, the son-in-law and his relatives should pay all the outstanding bridewealth before the deceased wife's relatives agree to perform the *kutara ruhahu*.

If the son-in-law has paid all the requested bridewealth, but had ill-treated his wife in any way, her relatives may ask for compensation before performing the ritual. Some Shona people take advantage of the fear of this type of *ngozi* to fleece the son-in-law. What complicates the matter is that the wife should be buried in the home cemetery of her husband, and if her relatives are not happy about anything, they may refuse to perform the marking of the grave ceremony. Since the corpse is in the home of the son-in-law, it becomes his burden to facilitate its burial as soon as possible. The *kutara ruhahu* ritual demands that one of the relatives of the wife takes the pick or hoe, and marks the spot on which the grave of his relative ought to be dug. The digging might be accompanied by words such as these, "My daughter, X, this is your new home in which you will rest in peace." After that ritual, other people, may begin the digging of the grave.

There are cases where some copses almost rot in mortuaries or at home before burial because the son-in-law and his relatives had failed to pay the demanded compensation. Usually the required compensation is so exorbitant that there is more injustice than justice in demanding it. The relatives of the dead woman use her death as their last leverage to obtain the outstanding bridewealth. Some people do this without willing to fulfill their responsibility of providing the son-in-law with a new wife who would take care of the remaining children or bear more children for her deceased sister. Once all the bridewealth is paid, the wife should fulfill her responsibility of bearing enough children, which she may not be able to do from the grave.

Some people argue that the families that refuse to perform the *kutara ruhahu* ritual would have been pushed by the deliberate neglect to pay bridewealth by some sons-in-law. In the past, if the son-in-law refused to pay bridewealth, the relatives of the wife would take her away from her marital home by force, and her husband would be compelled to pay the outstanding bridewealth. This phenomenon is known as *kubatira pfuma*. Nowadays, most parents have stopped doing that because most sons-in-law do not make any follow-up, and that may lead to divorce. Therefore, most relatives of the wife wait for the death of their daughter, so that they can claim the outstanding bridewealth before her burial. Usually, the extended family members of the son-in-law pool up resources to produce the required amount or number of cows.

Ngozi of an Aborted Fetus

Some Shona ethnic groups believe that the spirit of the aborted fetus can come back to haunt its mother because abortion is never justified among the traditional people of Zimbabwe. However, there are people who still do abortions for a variety of reasons. One of the popular causes of abortions in Zimbabwe is unplanned pregnancies of young girls, particularly in cases where the responsible father is refusing to marry the mother or take responsibility for the baby. Since it is illegal to perform abortions in Zimbabwe, some women may perform them secretly, despite the dangers of doing so. Because all life is sacred and should be protected, there is a general belief that some of the aborted babies' spirits would come back to haunt their mothers. Usually, these allegations surface when the woman gets married, and fails to conceive children. It is alleged that the failure to bear children by some married women may be the punishment by the spirits of the babies that they would have aborted in the past. It should be noted that the Shona know very well that not all women who fail to bear children would have performed an abortion at some point in their lives. In most cases, childlessness is a natural misfortune. It is believed that some women who abort babies prevent their spirits from coming back to haunt them by performing some rituals during the disposal of the fetus. They bury the aborted fetus along flowing rivers so that their spirits may calm down. The same burial place is used for premature babies. Although married couples can also perform abortion, it is very rare for a Shona couple to agree to abort a baby for any reason.

Placating *Ngozi*

All avenging spirits can be placated. Compensation for the wrong done should be paid, and its amount is determined by the nature and severity of the misdeed. Usually, the spirit of the deceased, through a traditional medical practitioner, charges the compensation. Once the compensation has been paid, the symptoms of the avenging spirit should cease. Unfortunately, those who would have died from the attacks by the avenging spirit cannot be brought back to life. The payment of the compensation is usually a family thing—family members of the perpetrator pool up resources to pay the family of the aggrieved spirit. There are two major reasons that force families to do this. First, in some cases, the perpetrator cannot afford to pay the demanded compensation alone. Second, the *ngozi* spirit attacks anybody who belongs to the extended family of the perpetrator. Usually, the actual perpetrator is spared by the *ngozi* until reparations are paid.

There are many methods of paying the compensation. It can be paid in cattle, goats, chicken, sheep, or money depending on the gravity of the offense. In most murder cases, about ten head of cattle are demanded. Many times, the payment of cattle is not convenient because of the place where the recipients live, hence, money is used. Those who live in urban areas might find it more conducive to be paid in cash instead of cattle. In that case, the compensation is charged in cattle, then translated to money. In the past, there were instances when *ngozi* spirits demanded wives from the families of their murderers. The spirit would demand a young girl who would be surrendered to the family of the deceased for marriage purposes. In some cases, that woman would not get married, but should remain the wife of the spirit. In other cases, the young brother of the deceased would marry the young girl to bear children for his dead brother. This form of compensation has been challenged in Zimbabwe because of the violation of the rights of the young girl who is used as compensation to a *ngozi* spirit without her consent. In most cases, the girl would be too young to give marital consent.

Among the Budjga of Mutoko, it was believed that one could avoid the *ngozi* of the person he would have murdered by performing a ritual soon after killing that person. One of the rituals was for the murderer to eat the *muputi/mutimwi* (waist string), the blood, flesh from the private parts of the deceased, his little fingers or toes, ears, tongue, or heart of the deceased.[7] This ritual may explain why most Karanga ethnic groups think that those people who die of the effects of witchcraft may not become *ngozi* because the witches, during their nocturnal cannibalistic feasts, perform *ngozi* sup-

---

7. Crawford, *Witchcraft and Sorcery in Rhodesia*, 88.

pressing rituals, as they devour their victim's flesh. However, very few Shona people who are not witches can be sadistic enough to cut the human flesh of the person that they would have killed. No sane Shona person except a witch may try to consume human flesh.

There are traditional medical practitioners who claim to have the expertise to exorcise *ngozi*, and this could be the only solution if the relatives of the *ngozi* refuse to accept compensation. M. L. Daneel, tapping from Kumbirai, says that a black goat or chicken was used for exorcising *ngozi*, and the ritual was performed under a *mushozhowa* tree, whose fruits are a delicacy to goats, or was carried out in the middle of a river or stream to cool down the angry spirit.[8] The relatives of the *ngozi's* reluctance to accept the compensation was a result of the vindictiveness of the *ngozi*. If the compensation cattle were not handled properly, and the right rituals meticulously performed, the *ngozi* could turn against its own people. The other reason for the rejection of the *ngozi* compensation is that some *ngozi* attacks happen several years after the murder or unjust event, and no one in the victim's family knows about it.

It is difficult to exorcise *ngozi* because it may be sent back by the relatives of the victim. Moreover, every family member of the affected must be involved in the rituals of exorcism. Everyone should eat the medicinal porridge called *svusvu*, and if any member of the family is excluded, the *ngozi* would attack him. In the end, family members clandestinely toss the avenging spirit back and forth among themselves. This tossing of the *ngozi* is called *kusundirana ngozi*, and is known to cause irreparable family divisions.

Becoming *Ngozi*

Some spirits may become avenging spirits on their own accord without any promptings from their living relatives. The Shona expect all the spirits of the people who are treated unjustly or killed either voluntarily or in accidents, to avenge their deaths. Their relatives do nothing but wait for the spirit of their ill-treated relative to avenge his death. If that does not happen as soon as the relatives expect, some relatives of the deceased may invoke the spirit of the dead so that it goes to seek justice. They do that by going to the grave of the deceased and offer tobacco or libation to the spirit, while instructing it to rise from the grave, and seek justice among the family members of the perpetrators.

Other people may visit a traditional medical practitioner so that they may be assisted in provoking the spirit of the dead to fight against the

---

8. Daneel, *Old and New in Southern Shona Independent Churches Vol. 1*, 139.

offenders. Some Shona ethnic groups immunize their children at birth, so that their spirits can become *ngozi* if they are murdered or ill-treated. Sometimes, relatives of the dead are believed to plant a tree called *mupfukwa* by the grave of the deceased. It is believed that at a certain stage of the tree's growth, each leaf that falls off the tree, would cause sickness, bad luck, or even death in the family of the wrong-doer. Sometimes many years pass-by without the offended spirit avenging its death. When it finally does, the victims might not know why they would be meeting such inexplicable misfortunes in their family. They usually consult a traditional medical practitioner, who advises them of the need to pay compensation to the relatives of the deceased, who in some cases, might not have any awareness of the murder being referred to, and for which they should receive compensation.

Symptoms of the *Ngozi* Spirit

There are several symptoms of the attack by the *ngozi* spirit. A family with members who experience recurring bad luck may suspect a *ngozi*. The bad luck may include but is not limited to the following: failure to get a job for which one is qualified, failure to get married after one has reached the marriageable age, barrenness, mental illness, being victimized by robbers, an insatiable desire to fight or cause harm to others, suicide, several unexplainable deaths in the family, and sicknesses that cannot be explained medically. This list does not imply that things will be alright and smooth all the time, but the avenging spirit is suspected if some of the misfortunes are bizarre and unfathomable. The Shona tolerate challenges, and accept natural explanations for those challenges, but they reach a point where they begin to believe that the causes of whatever bedevils them are spiritual.

There are reports of dead bodies that get swollen as soon as the person dies, to the extent that they may not fit in the coffin. Sometimes the body may fit in the coffin, but it becomes too heavy to lift. The grave may be difficult to dig. The perpetrator or any one of his family members may see the ghost of the killed person in dreams or apparitions. Some perpetrators are believed to hear voices of the deceased asking for the reason for which he was murdered. In some cases, the avenging spirit may possess one of the family members of the perpetrator to make known its needs. In addition to that, some kinds of illnesses are believed to be related to the avenging spirit. Mental illness is strongly believed to be connected to the avenging spirits. Most of the time, the Shona may suspect that their misfortunes are caused by an avenging spirit, although they might not be certain about it. Those with any reasonable suspicion of being attacked by *ngozi* may consult a traditional medical practitioner to have their fears or suspicions confirmed or disconfirmed.

Lessons

The fear of the avenging spirits has, to some extent, positively benefited the Shona people. It protects women from being abused by their own children. The belief in *ngozi* also teaches that life is sacred, and because of that it should not be taken away either intentionally or accidentally. Anyone who kills another person must accept responsibility by either paying restitution or facing the spiritual retribution. When someone is murdered, the whole community suffers, so the whole family of the perpetrator should be involved in the payment of the restitution. The Shona believe that no one can get away with murder even if it is committed secretly because the spirit of the dead will always come back to apprehend and punish the offender. The sooner the offender accepts responsibility over his actions, the lesser the misfortunes his family will encounter.

Christianity and *Ngozi*

The belief in *ngozi* has not received much criticism and condemnation from Christian missionaries as compared to ancestral veneration. One of the critical factors that may have led the Christian missionaries to remain relatively indifferent to the belief in *ngozi* could be the striking agreement between basic Christian teachings and the Shona moral teachings about the sacredness of human life. Both sides believe that life is sacred and is a priceless gift from the creator, hence it should be preserved at all costs. No human being should be deprived of life. Since no one knows with certainty when unborn babies become conscious human beings, both Christians and Shona people condemn abortion. Both Christians and the Shona people agree that no one has the authority to terminate another person's life even if that person is terminally ill. Life is not a private commodity of any individual; hence no individual may give it away or terminate it by suicide.

Despite some striking agreement between the Shona and Christian philosophy concerning the sacredness of life, Christianity permits the taking of human life in certain circumstances. Life can be taken away in an accident, and the perpetrator is exculpated. Life of a murderer, who has been convicted by the lawful courts of the land, can be terminated, if the judiciary system of the country deems it justifiable. In that case, the hangman is not accountable for taking the life of another person. The Shona see it from a different perspective. Killing another person in an accident, though understandable, should be accounted for by the one causing the death. They also believe that the hangman that carries out the wishes of the courts is accountable for the deaths of the people that he hangs. Whenever human blood is spilt, the one responsible for that should compensate the family of the deceased. It seems that the Christian churches qualify one of the Ten Commandments that says, *thou shall not kill*. The Shona do not exempt any one from observing the commandment that says, *thou shall not kill*. The missionaries might have found their teaching on the sacredness of human life a little bit deficient as compared to the Shona teachings.

Christianity teaches that human beings were created in the image of God, and because of that they deserve to be respected and treated with dignity. The Shona believe that there is nothing that violates the dignity of women more than an abusive son. Every son should love, respect, and care for his mother. Shona women may be victims of abuse from other people, but it is inconceivable to be a victim of one's own child. Any child who abuses his mother will be accountable to the spirit of the mother after her death. Christians see it differently. Abusers, like any other unrepentant sinners, will be sentenced to eternal suffering in hell.

There is also a striking similarity between Christianity and Shona Traditional Religion with regards to social teaching. Both groups base their social teaching on the Golden Rule of reciprocity that says that one should not do to others what he does not want to be done to him. One should not ill-treat the poor, the immigrant, and the marginalized. If one employs any one of them, he should be prepared to remunerate her justly. Children should respect their parents and never to neglect them in times of need. The slight difference between the two perspectives is that the Shona believe that anyone who ill-treats his parents, particularly his mother, or takes advantage of the vulnerability of the poor, will be accountable to the spirit of the affected person. Christians believe that the punishment and establishment of justice belongs to God alone. They also believe that all the evil-doers will be punished in hell. The Shona do not have the concept of the Christian hell.

The Shona and Christians differ on forgiveness. Both believe that transgressors of societal ethical codes can be forgiven if they repent. But for the Shona, transgressors of the societal moral standards may be forgiven if their repentance is real and accompanied by the payment of reparations. They believe that every attempt at reconciliation should be accompanied by restitution. The Shona realize that sending a murderer to jail may not bring food on the table of the family of his victim, but restitution does. Some Christians see it differently. A person can be forgiven after merely confessing his baneful deeds to a priest or pastor, and may not be required to pay compensation for the loss he would have caused.

The other striking similarity between Christian and Shona beliefs concerns life after death. Both groups believe that human life does not end with death, but it continues in the spiritual form. They believe that the dead can intercede for the living. The Christians call those people saints, and the Shona call them ancestors. However, the two groups differ concerning the nature of that life. For Christians, after death, the spirit of the dead waits for the day of judgment when God will reward the righteous with everlasting life in heaven, and eternally punish the evil-doers in hell. Some Christian groups believe that some good people go to be with God immediately after death. Such people become saints, who can intercede for the living before God. Some Christians believe that once a person dies, he ceases to have any power over the living, and he should wait for the day of judgment. Consequently, there is no spirit that has the power and authority to punish evil-doers. The Shona see it differently. Murdered people, exploited domestic workers, and ill-treated mothers do not wait for the day of judgment—they mete out their own punishment. They fight for justice. They have power to cause misfortunes in the families of perpetrators until compensation is paid. The God of Matonjeni was responsible for punishing evil-doers whose evil deeds affected the whole community, but he allowed other spirits to seek restitution for the injustice done. Furthermore, the Christian saints are in heaven, but the ancestors are in the homes of their relatives.

The Christian churches and African traditionalists differ concerning the dignity of women and their equality to men. Christians challenge the Shona traditionalists for using young girls as compensation for the *ngozi*. Human beings have a dignity that emanates from being created in the image of God, and should not be forced to marry persons that they do not love. To force a girl to marry someone is a gross violation of that girl's right to choose her own husband. The traditional Shona society did not feel the same. Although they acknowledged the inalienable rights of their daughters, they thought that the girls' rights could be overridden for the greater good. If the *ngozi* needed a wife as compensation, the Shona would sacrifice the girl for the happiness and continuity of the family. Where Christianity sees individual's human rights as inalienable, the Shona believe that every individual's rights are subordinate to the collective rights of the family and community. The individual can only be happy if the community is happy.

It seems that Christian missionaries failed to challenge the Shona belief in *ngozi*, and if they ever tried, they were not successful. Many Shona Christians hold both beliefs to be true. Most believe that the Christian God will judge the world at the end of time. They also believe that *ngozi* can punish evil-doers. They fear both hell and *ngozi*. Given the choice, most Shona people would want to avenge the injustice done to them, before they may surrender that right to God. Most Shona believers do not seem to see the contradiction in believing that a person can be in heaven, and be an avenging spirit at the same time. Most tend to forget the teaching of the Christian churches concerning the confession of sins and reconciliation. The Shona do not understand that once a murderer has been convicted and sentenced to a prison term, that is enough. For them, going to jail does not exculpate the wrongdoer of his offences, but the payment of compensation does.

Since some of the civil and customary laws of Zimbabwe have not been synchronized, some offenders are punished twice. They serve the jail sentence, and should also pay compensation to the family of the victim. Most Shona people have come to accept the importance of both punishments. Will the Shona reach a point where they stop being afraid of the avenging spirit? No. The fear of the avenging spirit is so pervasive and incapacitating that it will take a long time for the Shona to escape its grip. It seems that even the African clergy and pastors are also afraid of the avenging spirit, and will never discourage some of their family members from paying compensation for any injustice done. Some pastors attend funerals where the relatives of the deceased woman refuse to perform the necessary rituals, and most of them normally do not intervene. Most Christian churches in Zimbabwe do not have a theologically systematic response to the issue of *ngozi*. As of now, the deceased Shona people are not ready to surrender their inherited right to discipline evildoers to God. In fact, most Shona spirits are in no hurry to get to heaven, for they would rather become ancestors first before they can go to heaven.

6

Witchcraft

All people want to live a healthy, long, prosperous, and happy life. Unfortunately, most of the time, people's lives are full of challenges, such as sickness, untimely deaths, and poverty. These misfortunes remind humanity of its fragility, finitude, and the unpredictability of human life. Most people have come to accept these challenges as part of human life, although it is hard to understand why they happen. When misfortunes strike, human beings want to know their causes, so as to take appropriate measures to prevent them from happening again in the future. Although most causes of misfortunes are natural and physical, there are times when they are so weird, inexplicable, and unfathomable. These inexplicable and unfathomable causes of misfortunes have compelled Africans to believe in mysterious causes of misfortunes, such as witchcraft. Witchcraft is the belief in the possession of some mysterious, inherent, evil, and secret powers by some people, which they use to harm others.

Unlike in other parts of Africa, among the Shona of Zimbabwe, all kinds of witchcraft are considered evil. The person who claims or is believed to possess such powers is called a witch, if she is a woman, and a wizard, if he is a man. However, the Shona term, *muroyi*, which literally means witch, can be used for both men and women who employ witchcraft. Again, among the Shona, there is no distinction between witchcraft and a sorcery, and the distinctions that have been put forward by some scholars are primarily academic.[1] In this book, I will use the term witchcraft to refer to all kinds of mysterious evil employment, including what other scholars would term sorcery, because the ordinary Shona people do not make such a distinction.

There is no African religious practice that is as controversial and divisive as the practice of witchcraft. The early European settlers, anthropologists, missionaries, hunters, explorers, and fortune-seekers condemned the belief as superstitious. In Zimbabwe, the British South Africa Company administrators legislated The Witchcraft Suppression Act, Chapter 73 of

---

1. Chavhunduka, "Witchcraft and the Law in Zimbabwe," 129–47. In this article Chavhunduka argues for a distinction between a witch and a sorcerer, which he claims is absent in the The Witchcraft Suppression Act of 1899 that was enacted by the British South Africa Company that occupied Zimbabwe.

1899, which made it a criminal offence for anyone, including traditional medical practitioners, to name another person or him- or herself a witch, or to receive money as payment for identifying a witch.[2] In mainstream Christian churches, the official teaching about witchcraft is that it does not exist, although most members of such churches believe in the reality of witchcraft. African Independent Churches have made a big following because of their acceptance that witchcraft does exist. Most of them have incorporated healing sessions as part of their liturgy.

Is witchcraft a reality or a figment of the African's superstitious imagination? There is no consensus concerning the answers given for this question. Primarily, there are three schools of thought concerning the existence of witchcraft. The first school of thought argues that witchcraft is a reality whose existence can only be doubted by outsiders and those Africans whose minds have been tainted by the outsider's education. This group consists of Africans and some few outsiders. The second school of thought that comprises outsiders, some African members of the academia, and Christian churches argues that witchcraft is a figment of the African's imagination, and does not exist. A third school of thought consists of both Africans and outsiders who are indifferent. This group neither affirms nor denies the existence of witchcraft. One of the reasons for this controversy is the secrecy and mystery that surround the practice of witchcraft. It is only witches and traditional medical practitioners who claim to have the ability to see witches. The second reason for the controversy concerns the lack of empirical evidence concerning the efficacy of witchcraft. This lack of empirical evidence is characteristic of most religious beliefs that are espoused by the religious traditions of this world. The belief in witchcraft is not different from religious beliefs such as hell, heaven, karma, and God, because all cannot be empirically verified.

Types of Witchcraft

Night Witchcraft

First and foremost, among the Shona of Zimbabwe, unlike in West Africa, where witchcraft can be either good or evil, witchcraft is evil because its employment is done to harm others. For instance, in Ghana, the witchcraft spirit is considered neutral, and it takes its character from the way it is used by its host.[3] The Shona believe that witches are intrinsically evil be-

---

2. The Witchcraft Suppression Act (Chapter 73, 1899).
3. Abraham, "A Phenomenology of Witchcraft in Ghana," 53–66.

cause their devilish spells and nefarious activities can cause unimaginable misfortunes, such as bad luck, poverty, barrenness, illnesses, and untimely deaths to innocent people. To worsen the matter, witches bewitch unsuspecting people including children. In Zimbabwe, night witchcraft is the most feared practice because of the mysteries surrounding it. Most night witches are women, and are believed to have inherited their witchcraft from a parent or a member of the extended family.[4] Although some people occasionally confess to be witches, most people deny being witches even after being implicated by traditional medical practitioners. Their bewitching power is supposed to remain a mystery and secret. Night witches operate in the dark to prevent any detection by their victims. They attack people who are asleep. They can make themselves invisible, or may turn into animals during their nefarious operations. Their weirdness is compounded by their ability to enter locked doors without first unlocking them. This ability makes the people who believe in the existence of such a practice feel powerless and vulnerable. It is believed that night witches can travel for long distances on the back of familiars such as hyenas and crocodiles. They also tame and possess other animals and birds such as snakes and owls, that they may send on errands to harm their victims. During business hours, they are believed to walk around naked, which might be for the need of agility, weirdness, and avoidance of easy identification.

One of the most bizarre beliefs about night witches is that they lust for human flesh, and devour it whenever they kill someone. They are believed to hold hideous, nocturnal parties and macabre dancing orgies where they abominably desecrate graves by digging them up to get out human bodies, which they cook and eat. For the Shona, the eating of human flesh by witches is real, not symbolical, as Geoffrey Parrinder considers it to be the case among other African peoples who have a similar belief.[5] It is believed that each witch is scheduled to provide human flesh for the group, and failure to do that may be severely punished. One of the punishments is that the incompetent witch, who would have failed to provide human meat for the group when her turn to do so comes, might be compelled by the leader of the cabal to bewitch one of her own children or husband, so that the supply of human flesh remains constant. In such cases, it is dangerous to be a child or husband of a weaker witch.

Most Shona groups try to protect the bodies of their deceased from being devoured by the witches, by guarding the grave at night for a couple

---

4. Bourdillon, *The Shona Peoples*, 174.

5. Parrinder, *Witchcraft*, 149. For a comparative approach to witchcraft beliefs in Africa, the reader may read Parrinder's above-cited book, 132–49.

of days after the burial. Other Shona groups, particularly the Karanga of Masvingo, sweep clean the area surrounding the grave on the burial day, and sprinkle water on the dusty ground, so that the footprints of witches can be detected the following morning, if they try to desecrate the grave. It is believed that the witches have a magical whip that they get from a mysterious tree, which they use to open the grave by striking it in a ritualistic manner. They use the same stick to magically close the same grave after butchering the body of their victim. The families that have any reason to suspect that witches would have tempered with the graves of their deceased, usually consult a traditional medical practitioner, who then instructs them on how to appease the spirit of the violated dead person. The Shona never try to exhume the corpse to verify if the witches would have desecrated it because that would be a pernicious disrespect for the dead. Once one is buried, nobody has the authority to exhume his body unless it is required by the criminal law enforcement agents of the country.

Witches operate in cabals in which the most powerful witch becomes the leader. What E. E. Evans-Pritchard says about the Azande witches is equally true of the Shona witches: "witches usually combine in their destructive activities and subsequent ghoulish feasts. They assist each other in their crimes and arrange their nefarious schemes in concert."[6] Occasionally, some witches operate as individuals, but the norm is for them to combine their efforts. Although they act collectively, the members must be invited by one of the witches, who has a reason to bewitch a particular person. The members of the group need no other reason for bewitching somebody apart from being invited to do so by their colleague. If the bewitched person becomes sick or dies, it is the witch who would have invited others, who is more likely to be apprehended by the traditional medical practitioners. That same witch may be directly blamed for the misfortunes caused to the victim. One of the advantages that witches enjoy in working in groups is that even weaker witches can achieve their objectives through the intervention of their stronger colleagues.

The Shona believe that night witches operate in body and soul, which is different from West Africa, where witches' spirits are believed to leave their bodies on the bed as they attend organized meetings and bewitching errands.[7] Some Shona people also believe that the witches do not enter locked doors miraculously, but somebody, particularly the victim's ancestors, open the doors for them. They are believed to recite the totemic poems of the victim so that she unconsciously wakes up and opens the door for them. Once

---

6. Evans-Pritchard, *Witchcraft, Oracles, and Magic among the Azande*, 14.
7. Quarcoopome, *West African Traditional Religion*, 157.

inside the house, the witches are believed to cast a spell on the victim so that she does not wake up until they finish their fiendish activities, and are gone. Likewise, spouses whose partners are witches are placed under a spell that prevents them from waking up before their partners come back from their bewitching errands. These unfortunate spouses never wake up at night to find their spouses missing. Some witches are believed to leave one of their living-dead assistants known by the Karanga as *zvidhoma*, sleeping in their place to mislead the partner into believing that they are present.

It is believed that both men and women can be witches, although most witches are women. A male witch is believed to be hard-hearted, and once he bewitches someone, he is unlikely to reverse the effects of his witchcraft. However, the leader of the cabal is believed to be the most powerful woman, not the hard-hearted man. Witchcraft is one of the few areas where a woman's leadership is undisputed and highly valued. The male witch might be more useful in orgiastic feasts that the witches are believed to hold, where he is alleged to engage in ritualistic sex with the leader of the group, but he is not the leader, and does not make decisions for the cabal.

The Shona believe that the witches also employ the use of some spirits, which are called *zvidhoma*. *Zvidhoma* are the spirits of some of the young people that witches resuscitate from the grave after death, so that they can train them as their own spiritual children. Geoffrey Parrinder describes *zvidhoma* as the spirits of the newly dead that are captured by witches on their way to the spirit world, and are turned into frightening ghosts.[8] These *zvidhoma* are invisible to the public but are treated as human beings by the witches who own them. They are believed to eat human food, and partake in the orgiastic and ghoulish night feasts with their *mothers* and *fathers*. During years of drought when food is scarce, it is believed that *zvidhoma* are sent by their mothers and fathers to eat food in other people's homes without their hosts' knowledge. If a woman observes that her family consumes an unimaginable large quantity of food, she may suspect the involvement of the uninvited and invisible guests—*zvidhoma*. As I was growing up in my rural village under Chief Nyajena, the solution would be to add salt to all the food, since it was believed that *zvidhoma* were allergic to salt. *Zvidhoma* are believed to include both females and males, and some of them may get married to each other. Their parents give them human names by which they may identify themselves after beating up someone. They usually talk through their victim after the traditional medical practitioner uses incense (*rukata*) to cast them out. However, in most cases, *zvidhoma* refuse to reveal

---

8. Parrinder, *Witchcraft: European and African*, 133.

their names and the names of their senders even under serious interrogation by the sacred inquisitors.

Zvidhoma either frighten or beat up their victims. Whatever they choose to do, the effect will be the same. The victim becomes sick, and sometimes starts hallucinating and seeing things that other people do not see. Usually, the victim gets into a trance and begins to speak using the voice of the *chidhoma*. Once that happens, the family of the victim may burn incense that is known as *rukata* to exorcize the victim. Sometimes the *zvidhoma* may temporarily leave the victim, but they may come back again for the same victim. The Shona are not quite agreed as to how *zvidhoma* frighten or beat up their victims. Some Karanga groups believe that *zvidhoma* have shadows that they may use during operations by casting them into contact with the victim's shadow. It is believed that the contact between the shadows is extremely dangerous, and may cause serious illness or the death of the victim. Some Shona groups believe that *zvidhoma* beat up their victims, as if in a boxing arena.

Night witchcraft can be inherited from one's own relatives, particularly one's mother or grandmother. Ordinarily, witchcraft is passed on to a kid when she is still too young to resist, and before she is mature enough to have any recollection of her acceptance of the shameful trade. Sometimes the bewitching inheritance is passed on to the daughter or son after the express acceptance of the inheritor, who then is given the bewitching concoctions and other paraphernalia. If mature enough, the inheritor must undergo training on how to operate as a witch. Most Shona people suspect that a witch's daughters are also witches, although that has been proved not to be always the case. The witch might not pass on her trade to all her daughters, but just one who she thinks has a disposition that is suitable for the trade. Women who are sulky, mean, selfish, and pugnacious may be associated with witchcraft.

Night witchcraft can also be gotten from a person who is not related to the receiver. The Karanga believe that a woman who is interested in becoming a witch may approach a well-known witch in the community so that she can receive bewitching training. This training is initiated by an incision that is made on the navel or back of the trainee, on which some medicine is rubbed. The Karanga call this type of acquisition of witchcraft *kutemegwa uroyi*. Of course, this way of passing on witchcraft can also be used by the woman's immediate family member. It is believed that this type of witchcraft acquisition can be reversed provided the recipient has not consumed human flesh. Once human flesh is consumed, the acquisition becomes consummated, and almost irrevocable.

The Shona believe that night witchcraft can be a result of the witch being possessed by the spirit of a relative or stranger who was a witch. This spirit is known as *mamutsamurimo*. Usually, the bewitching spirit does not seek permission to possess its host, but it imposes itself on its host. The chosen person may begin to bewitch people without having the knowledge of her evil and loathsome actions. Some women may have dreams in which they act like witches, and that may make them aware of their unconscious bewitching errands. These witches do not choose to be evil but they are compelled by the bewitching spirits to participate in bewitching activities. Despite being involuntary witches, they are still detested just like any other kind of witches. Some hosts of such bewitching spirits realize that they are witches after being apprehended by a traditional medical practitioner. Some Shona groups believe that the bewitching spirit can be exorcized, unlike the inherited witchcraft. However, there is a strong belief that if the witch has already eaten human flesh, then her witchcraft cannot be exorcized. What some traditional medical practitioners can do is to try to lessen the severity of one's witchcraft by inducing vomiting in her, which is believed to get rid of the human flesh that one would have consumed. This medical procedure is known as *kurutsisa*.

Agricultural Witchcraft

The Shona call agricultural witchcraft *divisi*. This type of witchcraft allows the owner to increase his harvest by using evil and mysterious ways. *Divisi* is a preserve of men, perhaps because in the past, only men owned the land. The agricultural witchcraft can be employed in several ways. Some *divisi* witches are believed to possess some mysterious powers that enable them to wake up other villagers at night so that they come to the witch's fields in which they work semi-consciously throughout the night. The victims might dream of their ordeal or might wake up the following morning feeling very tired. The *divisi* witch may possess a python that lives in one of his granaries, and is used to collect crops mysteriously from other farmers' fields. Some *divisi* witches are believed to own thousands of ants that they may send to collect undissolved fertilizer grains from their neighbors' farms. The ants then bring that fertilizer and deposit it onto the witch's crops. *Divisi* is considered witchcraft because it is practiced secretly, and may cause the death of other villagers through starvation if they fail to harvest enough crops to feed their families. It is also believed that some *divisi* witches perform incestuous rituals in their fields to increase the power of their *divisi*. Incestuous relationships strongly offend the ancestors who may withhold the rain from the whole community as punishment for its commission. This type of witchcraft can be passed on to one's sons and grandsons.

Sexual Witchcraft

Sexual witchcraft is popularly known as *mubobobo*, and is one of the most bizarre types of witchcraft among the Shona. People who own this type of witchcraft can have sexual encounters with members of the opposite sex, mysteriously and secretly, without the consent of their victims. Both men and women may possess *mubobobo*, but the majority of *mubobobo* witches are men. These men visit their victims either at night or during the day, and engage in mysterious and non-consensual sexual activities with them. The victims do not see the witch but may have vivid experiences of the witch's wicked actions. Sometimes the targeted women see the *mubobobo* man in a dream, but when they wake up, they only find signs of a normal sexual activity such as semen. These witches enter locked doors mysteriously, and cast a spell on the husband or wife of the victim so that he or she remains asleep until they finish their sinister activities.

If the *mubobobo* man victimizes a pregnant woman, it is believed that she loses the baby through a miscarriage. However, *mubobobo* men are believed not to have the ability to impregnate their victims, or even pass on sexually transmitted infections. Women who live in the village in which the *mubobobo* man resides, know his identity because some of them would have had sexual encounters with him in their dreams. Among the Zezuru, it is believed that a *mubobobo* man may not be able to violate a woman unless he manages to perform some rituals that involve his victim prior to his visit. It is believed that if a *mubobobo* man shakes a woman's hand during the day as a way of greeting, he may use the same hand to cast a spell on that particular woman so that when he visits her at night, she opens the door for him and cooperates with his evil doings. These witches are depraved because they violate unsuspecting people and may cause miscarriages in pregnant women.

Love Witchcraft

The Shona call the love potion, *mupfuwira*, and is used by women to enhance the quality of their husbands' love. This type of witchcraft is believed to be added to the food of a promiscuous or abusive husband, who then consumes it, and has his behavior changed.[9] It is also believed that even faithful and good husbands can be victims of *mupfuwira*. This witchcraft can alter the mental status of the victim to the extent where he behaves like a zombie. Such victims can be identified by their refusal to associate and socialize with other men outside the home. They follow their wives wherever they go. They may as well perform household chores that are traditionally assigned to women such as washing nappies, cooking, and bathing kids. Some of *mupfuwira* men are abused by their wives. These witches may get involved in extra-marital affairs with the knowledge of the husbands, who do nothing to stop that behavior. Some victims become so docile that they fail to make any decisions without the express authorization by their wives. Although this scenario may not be interpreted as a consequence of *mupfuwira* by modern Shona men and women, in the traditional Shona society, there was a clear division of labor that was not expected to be violated. The contemporary Shona society encourages men and women to assist each other in the home, but some domestic chores have remained gender sensitive.

The most famous kind of *mupfuwira* is the *chipotanemadziro*, which is produced from a lizard that frequents the hut in which food is cooked. The *chipotanamadziro* (lizard) is killed and its flesh is mixed with other bodily fluids such as menstrual blood and mucus, and then clandestinely applied to the husband's food. Once consumed, the man is supposed to behave like a lizard, hovering around the kitchen like a zombie. Among the Shona, the round hut kitchen is a place for women and ancestors. Some men believe that *mupfuwira* has no effect on them because they sense its presence in the food, and may refuse to eat it. If they eat the food, they may vomit it, which makes the witchcraft ineffective. Some people have argued that *mupfuwira rudo* (love potion is love), an assertion that has been disputed by others who believe that sometimes the effects of *mupfuwira* are fatal. If the quest for love turns the beloved into a docile, gullible, indecisive, exploitable, and lethargic zombie, then, it is not good.

Property Protection Witchcraft

The property protection witchcraft is known by the Shona as *rukwa*. *Rukwa* is used to protect one's properties from thieves and vandals. Whoever steals food, animals, or property to which the medicine has been applied is affected in one way or another. First, the victim might be forced to return the stolen goods by a mysterious voice that keeps reminding him to return the property to its owner. Second, the stolen property might stick to the

---

9. Rodlach, *Witches, Westerners, and HIV*, 89.

thief's hands until the thief is apprehended and the witchcraft reversed. Third, if the *rukwa* is in the food that has been consumed, whatever would have been eaten would start crying in the belly of the thief. For instance, a stolen goat may begin to make noise in the belly of the thief. Sometimes, the thief's belly permanently enlarges. At times the victimized thieves die because of *rukwa*.

Strangers to the Shona traditional values and morality might not see how *rukwa* can be said to be witchcraft. First of all, the Shona society believe that no one should be denied food when in need. Therefore, sojourners can just sit in any field and enjoy water melons or sugarcane if they are hungry, and that is not considered stealing. However, the application of *rukwa* to one's fields deprives hungry people of food. The other factor that makes *rukwa* some kind of witchcraft is that the owner should have antidotes to reverse its effects, which should be done as soon as possible to prevent the death of the thief. In some cases, the witch fails to reverse the effects of *rukwa*, and the thief may end up dying. So, *rukwa* is anti-social, and a result of selfishness and individualism that were never a characteristic of the communal life.

Poisoning

Some witches have the knowledge of poisonous herbs that can be used to poison unsuspecting people. The Shona call this type of witchcraft *kudyisa*. Both men and women may use this type of witchcraft. The poison is applied to the food or drink of the unsuspecting victim. Men who use this witchcraft are believed to place it in the beer mug, which is then consumed by the targeted person. The Shona are so afraid of being poisoned to the point that whoever brings a beer mug to another person, must take a sip first, then hands it to the one who wants to drink it. This taking of a sip is called *kubvisa uroyi* (removing witchcraft). In the modern times, some witches are believed to use arsenic dip or other poisonous chemicals that are used in agriculture. This type of witchcraft is very dangerous. Some scholars, such as Gordon Chavhunduka, argue that the existence of this type of witchcraft has some more credibility than the other types whose existence he seems to downplay as superstitious and mythological.[10]

10. Chavhunduka, "Witchcraft and the Law in Zimbabwe."

Muposo/Chitsinga

Muposo or *chitsinga* may be translated as trap witchcraft, and is mainly employed by men. It is believed that such men acquire this type of witchcraft from witches who live in an imaginary place called Maroro. The Karanga also believe that *muposo* can be acquired in Chipinge, one of Zimbabwe's eastern cities. The acquisition of this witchcraft is known as *kuromba*. This witchcraft can be buried in the ground along the path that is used by the intended victim. That is why some modern researchers have nicknamed it, *landmine* because it is supposed to work like one. It works only after being detonated by the victim, who unintentionally steps on it. Once stepped on, the victim can be paralyzed immediately. The victim might also suffer from a serious headache. *Muposo* acts suddenly. It can also affect people for whom it was not intended. That is why Shona people are very careful when they use paths, particularly crossroads. Many traditional medical practitioners say that it is very difficult to reverse the effects of *muposo*.

Lightning

Some Shona people are believed to possess the lightning witchcraft. These witches are believed to be able to control lightning (*mheni*), and cause it to strike a particular person or place. It is widely believed that this type of witchcraft is popular in Manicaland, one of the provinces in Zimbabwe. There are two types of lightning witches. The first type is believed to be able to manufacture clouds even outside the rain season so that they can produce lightning that would strike their intended victim. The second type is less dangerous because such witches have to wait for the coming of the rain season so that they can send the lightning to strike their victims. They wait for a conducive environment, which they cannot create themselves. This wait gives the intended victim an opportunity to reconcile with the witch before the rain season arrives. It also allows the witch to change his mind because of the passage of time. Some lightning witches have been heard threatening their intended victims by saying, "I will deal with you during the rainy season." However, it should be noted that the above statement can be used by anybody to scare off his enemies.

There is a story that widely circulated in the newspapers in Zimbabwe in the 1980s that had something to do with a lightning witch who approached a certain police station in one of the rural areas of Zimbabwe. He is reported to have told the police officers that he was tired of being a lightning witch, and had brought his paraphernalia so that the officers would help him destroy them. It is said that the officers made fun of him, and asked him to prove that his witchcraft was authentic. He did. Within a couple of minutes there was a small dark cloud hovering above the police station, and a bolt of lightning struck the sole tree that was in the compound. The officers were dumbfounded and chased the man away from the station.

Chikwambo

Chikwambo is a malicious and frightful gnome that is primarily used by the witches to enrich themselves. The *chikwambo* can be in the form of a mysterious small person who sometimes appears to some selected people. It may also be in the form of a medicinal horn that has blood and other concoctions inside it. It is believed to be able to steal money from other people, and enrich its owner in other ways. The *chikwambo* becomes problematic when it demands the blood of one of the relatives of the owner. Once in a while, the *chikwambo* mysteriously kills a relative of its owner for blood. If the *chikwambo* is in the form of a mysterious person, it may harass one of the daughters of the owner demanding sexual favors from her. The biggest challenge with *chikwambo* is that it is difficult, or almost impossible to get rid of, even if the owner no longer requires its services. The traditional medical practitioners who claim to have the power to kill *zvikwambo* are scarce and very expensive. Whoever acquires a *chikwambo* should know that he is in for a long-lasting association with it. Its possession by one of the family members causes unrepairable divisions in the family.

Reasons for Bewitching

The most widespread reason for bewitching people is the insatiable lust for human flesh that witches do have. It is believed that human flesh makes them more powerful, fearsome, and healthier. They are believed to hold meetings at the graveyards at night at which they feast on human flesh. Witches also bewitch people because they want to retaliate for an evil done to them or to one of their family members. Sometimes people who get offended cannot retaliate in any physical way because they may not be strong enough to physically fight the offender. Some offended persons might not want to fight the offender because of the fear of violating the law. For some Africans, the only way one can take revenge for a wrong done, without being held accountable for the offence, is by bewitching the offender.

It is also believed that some people bewitch others because of jealousy. They may envy their homes, cows, children, or jobs. They may bewitch their neighbors to impoverish them. It has also been argued that some people are anti-social. They just want to see other people suffering. They just hate to see them happy. Some witches do it for the sake of doing it. They possess the witchcraft and they feel that they should use it. However, it is believed that most witches are provoked into action by the tension between them and their victims. Hence, most victims of witchcraft are people who live in the same neighborhood with the witch.

Protection

For most African people witchcraft is a reality, which must be feared, and from whose effects people must protect themselves. As a means of protection, some people use charms and armlets that are believed to ward off witches and their collaborators. Sometimes people dig in medicinal pegs into all paths that lead into their homes. These pegs are believed to make it difficult for witches to enter the protected home. In addition to the medicinal pegs, incense (*rukata*) may be burnt in a broken clay pot (*chaenga*) and is placed on all paths that lead into the home. Some African people believe that prevention is better than cure, so, they engage traditional medical practitioners in exposing witches through witch-hunting. These controversial and largely unorthodoxy traditional medical practitioners, who are also known as *vana tsikamutanda,* move from one village to another, exposing witches and exorcizing them of their witchcraft. Some African Independent Churches also sprinkle holy water in the homes of their followers as a way of preventing witches and evil spirits from entering.

There is also another type of exposition of witches that is done by performing what the Shona people call *bembera,* which means accusing somebody of witchcraft indirectly, and persuading or demanding that witch to withdraw his baneful effects from the sick person.[11] Suppose somebody is very sick in the village, the members of the sick person's family might consult a traditional healer, who may identify the witches causing the sickness. The head of the sick person's family, with the assistance of the village head, may gather all the villagers at their normal meeting place. At that gathering, the head of the sick person's family is supposed to tell all the people about the illness of their family member if they did not know about it already. He is also expected to let them know of the family's awareness of the identity of the witch.

He may go on to threaten the witch, and give him a deadline to reverse the effects of the witchcraft. It is believed that after the meeting, the

---

11. Crawford, *Witchcraft and Sorcery in Rhodesia*, 267.

witches are supposed to secretly give the sick person some antidote that is likely to restore her health. This application of an antidote is known as *kuworonora*, which means to withdraw the witchcraft. No witch is expected to refuse to give heed to a call to withdraw her witchcraft after a *bembera* is performed.[12] However, some witches are believed to ignore the *bembera* until the sick person dies.

Another way of protecting oneself from the effects of witchcraft is to live amicably with one's neighbors. The people who quarrel a lot with their neighbors, and do not respect them are likely to attract the full wrath of the witches. One should respect her neighbors because any disrespect towards them might attract retaliation through witchcraft. Avoiding being boastful is another way of evading the attention of witches. One should be humble, shunning all boastfulness concerning one's wealth and achievements. There was a time when people would not eat food that other villagers did not have for the fear of making witches jealousy. Kids who herd cows should make sure that they do not stray and destroy other people's crops because that is likely to attract the wrath of witches. When about to embark on a journey, one should not let the neighbors know about it because they might bewitch him during the trip.

Some people try to protect their families from witchcraft to no avail. Some of them migrate (*kutama*) to distant villages to escape the reach of the witches. Some people change their jobs so that they can be away from the people who they suspect to be witches. It is believed that witches do not pursue their victims if they move away to resettle elsewhere. The migration of the victim or her family shows that the victim has accepted defeat, and should not be pursued. This migration also pacifies the situation since witchcraft usually thrives in environments of hatred, jealous, and quarrels. Moving away puts an end to the situations that create animosity. A witch's own children may also run away from their bewitching parent and resettle elsewhere.

Some people who have moved away for resettlement to have a fresh start claim that their fortunes have changed for the better. Most of the misfortunes that would have been bedeviling them just disappear as soon as they move away. However, some people who have moved away from their troublesome villages claim to have not experienced any change of fortune. In fact, some people have experienced worse misfortunes in their new homes than they did in their original homes. Consequently, some have gone back to their original homes. Sometimes, only the sick person is moved to a different home, and this is called *kusengudza*. *Kusengudza* is an indication

---

12. Evans-Pritchard, *Witchcraft, Oracles, and Magic among the Azande*, 33–34.

that the witch causing the illness lives in the same home or neighborhood. It can also be an indication that the witch would have set up his harmful medicines in the home of the sick person, and for her to recuperate, she has to be moved to another home that is free from the nefarious medicines and spells of the witch.

Some people do not try to appease witches in any other way, for they retaliate (*kudzorera*). Once they identify the witch who is causing their misfortunes, and try to protect themselves to no avail, they visit a traditional medical practitioner, who gives them some medicines that can ricochet the spells back to the witches. Whatever evil thing that is intended for the victim, backfires, and attacks the family of the witch. The efficacy of this type of protection lies in the power of the protective medicines used. The use of any weaker protective medicines has disastrous consequences. More often than not it frustrates the witch and compels him to use more powerful witchcraft, or to solicit for more help from more powerful witches. Although there are some people who argue that this retaliation is justified, other people think that it makes the victim a witch, just like the perpetrator. Such retaliation is believed to cause death and unexplainable misfortunes to the innocent relatives of the witch. The Shona believe that the killing of anybody even by accident is never allowed.

This line of argument may be unpersuasive to an outsider who believes that if an intruder enters his home in an attempt to harm him or any member of his family then he is justified to use reasonable force to defend himself or his family. That reasonable force may be the use of a gun to shoot the intruder. For the traditional Shona, life is sacred, and should never be taken away for any reason. So, the *kudzorera* is not intended to cause any harm to the witch or his family, but to warn him to ceasefire. If the retaliation causes the death of one of the witch's family members then whoever is retaliating has also become a witch.

Most Shona people teach their children from a tender age not to eat food from other people's homes without first obtaining explicit permission from their parents or guardians. This unrestrained eating of food from other people's homes is called *kukwata*. The kid is told, "*Usadya kumaraini, unoroyiwa*," which literally means, do not eat at the neighbors' homes because you will be bewitched. The predominant reason for educating one's kids about *kukwata* is the fear of witchcraft, particularly witchcraft that can be laced onto one's food by the witch. Since people do not know the identity of the witch, all neighbors including relatives are suspects. This discipline should be imparted on the kids because the Shona believe that food should be shared with everyone who needs it, hence, children will be offered food by relatives and strangers frequently. It is a disgrace not to offer food to other people, and the people who are offered the food should accept it. But when adults accept food, they are usually alert to ensure that no poison would have been laced on the food. Since kids do not have the wisdom to inspect the food for witchcraft, they should rather refuse the food that is offered to them by their neighbors.

The Shona have a method of testing for witchcraft in liquids. If it is beer or other traditional drinks, the one offering them should take a small sip before handing the drink to the other person. This ritual is done to provide evidence that the drink is not harmful in any way. Traditionally, the guest is encouraged to share his meal with one of the family members of the host as a guarantee that the food is free from witchcraft. Adults are not expected to deny the food that they are offered by their neighbors because the denial might be interpreted as an accusation of witchcraft. The Shona know that the witches may take advantage of the innocence of the kids, and then bewitch them. Consequently, the commandment to one's kids is simply, "Don't accept food from the neighbors."

Witchcraft: Fiction or Reality?

There is no agreement on this issue. There are two schools of thought that have put forward their arguments for the existence and non-existence of witchcraft. On the one hand, one school of thought argues that witchcraft is a reality whose existence should never be doubted. It is real and dangerous. It causes a lot of misfortunes to innocent people. This group consists of conservative insiders, particularly Africans. On the other hand, another school of thought argues that witchcraft does not exist. It is a figment of the African's fictitious and superstitious imagination. Both schools of thought claim to have evidence to support their diametrically opposed perspectives.

Let us look at the insiders' arguments first. Insiders argue that the belief in witchcraft is very widespread in Africa. Millions of Africans believe that witchcraft is a reality, and all those people cannot be wrong. Even in Europe, there was a time when they believed in the existence of witchcraft, and had it not been for their barbaric and horrendous way of dealing with witches, the belief could still be existing in Europe today. In the West, the remnant of such beliefs can be witnessed in some of their movies, and holidays such as Halloween. Of course, Africans, just like any other religious people of this world, may have exaggerated some of the baleful activities of the witches, here and there, but that does not render all their beliefs about witchcraft to be erroneous. Some of the Africans, who believe in the existence of witchcraft must have experienced something that convinces them about its existence.

To argue that witchcraft does not exist is to demean and trivialize the collective intelligence and experiences of the African peoples.

The other piece of evidence that has been put forward in support of the reality of witchcraft concerns the affirmations of traditional medical practitioners. These traditional medical specialists tell people that witchcraft exists, therefore, it does exist. The traditional medical practitioners possess special knowledge about spiritual and mysterious things that witches do in secret. Like Western medical practitioners, traditional medical practitioners are specialists in their areas of influence. They have no plausible reason to mislead the whole continent. Africans trust these experts, just as Westerners trust their medical practitioners. If a Western medical doctor tells a patient that his sickness is caused by a particular issue, the patient believes him because he knows that he has a special knowledge in diseases, their causes, and remedies. The same should be applied to African traditional healers. They too are true experts in their respective fields, and what they say should be respected. Believers in Western medicines may seek a second opinion from a different doctor, and most of the time, the same diagnosis is given. Africans do the same; if they do not agree with a sacred practitioner's diagnosis of a particular disease, they are free to have a second opinion. In addition to that, those in need of medical attention, visit traditional medical practitioners living in distant areas, and who have no prior knowledge of the patient, his family, and the social conflicts that may have provoked the witches.

Moreover, some people, without duress, testify that they are witches, and their testimonies should not be doubted. J. R. Crawford, in his 1967-book, *Witchcraft and Sorcery in Rhodesia*, compiled several witchcraft confessions from the records of the Attorney General of Zimbabwe, the then Rhodesia. Some of these confessions are believable. Some of the confessions come from the late Petros' wife, Sarah, Betty, and Madora, all of chief Chehudo. Sarah confessed that she had acquired witchcraft from Betty, and had recruited Madora to become a witch. Together, they claimed to have bewitched Sarah's husband, Petros, who then died. They again claimed to have bewitched Madora's baby who also died at Sarah's home because she refused to give some antidote to the baby. In retaliation, Madora is then believed to have hit and killed Sarah's child with a log.[13] The testimonies that the three women gave were strikingly similar, and very convincing.

Furthermore, some people claim to have bewitched and killed other people including their own children.[14] Most of the confessing witches

---

13. Crawford, *Witchcraft and Sorcery in Rhodesia*, 45–49. All the names I have used are fictitious. The real names that Crawford uses can be found in his book.

14. Read Parrinder, *Witchcraft*, 161–65, for some confessions by witches

claim to have devoured the flesh of their victims in their nocturnal feasts. The confessors usually name other witches with whom they operate, and give detailed narratives of how they acquired their witchcraft, and ply their business. They sometimes reveal the reason for which they would have bewitched their victims. Some witches, after being exposed, agree to reverse the effects of their baneful influence, and in some cases, the sick person recovers. Some witches expose their bewitching paraphernalia for the traditional medical practitioners and the members of the public to see and destroy. If these people were not real witches, they would not have any bewitching concoctions.

In addition to that, to be a witch is not a desirable thing in Africa, particularly, after one has been exposed. In some African cultures, witchcraft accusation can lead to someone's embarrassment, ostracization, divorce, or death. Claiming to be a witch is not something that makes a person proud. In fact, confessing to be a witch dehumanizes the confessor. It is embarrassing, not only to the one confessing, but also to her family. It affects the prospects of her children in marriage. No one wants her daughter or son to marry a person whose mother or father is a well-known witch, particularly the one who professes witchcraft publicly. Considering the severe consequences of confessing to be a witch, no one may willingly testify that she is a witch unless it is true. It would be like an innocent person confessing to be a murderer with full awareness of the possible consequences. Perhaps, there might be a few innocent people who confess to be murderers because of one reason or another, but most of the confessed murderers are real.

Another reason is that there are many mysterious and inexplicable illnesses that continue to dumbfound Western medical practitioners in Africa. "Occasionally deaths have occurred for which the western medicine could find no other explanation than that the patient himself to be bewitched."[15] In Zimbabwe, there are instances where patients are told by the physicians that there is nothing wrong with them, although they claim to be sick. Some patients have been advised by their physicians to try *chivanhu* (traditional healing methods), which means that the patient has to try alternative medicines. Sometimes sick people claim to see things that other people do not see, and the Shona believe what they see to be *zvidhoma*. Some patients who are not supposed to die from their ailments, end up dying, to the greatest disillusionment of the attending physicians. There are also patients who would have failed to heal in hospital who are reported to have been healed by traditional medical practitioners. Yes, some patients do not respond to traditional medical interventions—they die, but patients die in Western

---

15. Bourdillon, *The Shona Peoples*, 173.

hospitals as well. Both Africans and Christians believe that life comes from God, and the physician is merely an instrument of God. The death of a patient in the care of a physician does not mean that the physician's diagnosis and interventions were erroneous.

Also, belief in the existence of witchcraft can be compared to the Christian beliefs in heaven, hell, demons, Satan, angels, and other heavenly entities. There is no single person who has been to heaven or hell, so that he can cogently and experientially explain where these places are and how they look like. No one has ever seen Satan or demons, face to face. What Christians do is to believe what is written in their scriptures and traditions. The testimonies of their patriarchs and matriarchs give them the evidence that their beliefs are true. Although their beliefs do not quite make sense to an outsider, Christians have the right to believe in what they believe. The fact that no one has ever been to heaven or hell, or has seen Satan or demons, does not necessarily prove that they do not exist. The same should be applied to the belief in witchcraft. It is a mystery that cannot be fully comprehended by outsiders, and that does not necessarily mean that witchcraft does not exist. All belief systems should be tested by the same fire, if that is the only way they can be proved to be real or not.

On the other hand, the opposing school of thought argues that witchcraft does not exist. Most of the people who belong to this group are outsiders, some educated Africans, and some members of the mainline churches. This group argues that the illness that is thought to be induced by witchcraft is a result of telepathy. Some people have stronger minds than others. The psychologically stronger can cause harm to others by wishing them to suffer, and when that happens, they then believe that they are witches.[16] Sometimes those who confess to be witches do it because of guilty conscience. If someone wished ill-luck for another person, and if by coincidence that person falls sick or encounters a misfortune, the wisher of ill-luck may feel guilty, and may end up confessing to be a witch.[17]

Another reason that has been put forward to reject the existence of witchcraft is that the accusations of witchcraft follow a pattern of tension and conflict in society. Usually one accuses his pronounced enemies in situations such as polygamy, work places, and politics.[18] Witches are identified among one's neighbors and relatives because they are the people with whom one interacts. Most Africans repress hostility, frustration, and

---

16. Quarcoopome, *West African Traditional Religion*, 157.
17. Ibid., 157.
18. Evans-Pritchard, *Witchcraft, Oracles, and Magic among the Azande*, 45.

anxiety, which may find expression in witchcraft accusations.[19] There is so much hostility in the human society, and most of it is repressed because of the need to maintain peace and harmony. Some people are very frustrated because of their failures, and some evil things that other people do to them. Some end up venting out their hostility by accusing others of witchcraft. Accusing others of witchcraft enables them to hate the so-called witches without being blamed for being anti-social, which is one of the recipes of being accused of witchcraft.

In addition to that, sometimes the people who request the service of a traditional healer to identify a witch may influence the healer to pick out the person that they believe to be the witch. In some case, when people go to consult a traditional medical practitioner, they already have suspects, particularly those people with whom they have quarreled or disagreed. Usually, the healer does not directly identify the witch, but he merely gives hints. In those cases, the relatives of the sick person, usually name the witch themselves because they already have someone in their minds. Suspicion falls on those who have motives to bewitch others. If the healer names a witch that the relatives of the sick person never suspected of witchcraft because she is their friend, they may disagree with the medical practitioner, and would refuse to pay for his services. They may also destroy his reputation by telling their neighbors that *n'anga iyi haivoni* (this traditional medical practitioner is not authentic).

Some anthropologists have argued that witchcraft is the way Africans try to explain the misfortunes that they encounter in life. There is so much misfortunes in the world. There is sickness, death, bad luck, poverty, and so on. These misfortunes are always present, and are sometimes recurrent. It is very intriguing for people that some of these misfortunes have no logical explanations. Why does lightning strike one person, and leave others in the same room untouched? In the case of a car accident, why do some people die, and others survive? Why do some people get jobs while others do not, even when they are better qualified for the same jobs? Sometimes it is not easy to understand why things go wrong.[20] When Africans look at these misfortunes, they see an evil power that drives the misfortunes. That power is witchcraft. "When misfortunes are overwhelming, inexplicable, irrational, they are attributed to witchcraft."[21] However, these misfortunes may have natural causes, which scientific methods may not be able to explain adequately at that moment.

19. Shorter, *African Culture and The Christian Church*, 140.
20. Bourdillon, *Religion and Society*, 188.
21. Shorter, *African Culture and the Christian Church*, 139.

Furthermore, one of the most common beliefs about witchcraft is that a person may be a witch without being conscious of that fact. Since witchcraft can be practiced without the knowledge of the witch, no one can successfully defend herself if accused of practicing witchcraft.[22] One of the reasons that prevents some witches to know that they are witches is that they are possessed by bewitching spirits during their activities. They only go on bewitching errands when they are under the influence of the spirit. Many of the possessed witches are believed to have no knowledge of their dangerous activities, so they may not refute the accusations. If you are accused of witchcraft, it does not help trying to deny it because you might not have the knowledge. Once accused of witchcraft, then you are a witch. Ignorance is no defense. There is no valid defense that one can put up for her innocence. Many people might confess that they are witches to confirm what other people are saying about them. "Since you say that I am a witch, therefore, I must be one."

Moreover, male bias has also been noted in witchcraft accusations. As has been said above, the majority of witches are women. Once one has been accused of being a witch, that person loses her dignity and humanity. A witch is anti-social, and the fact that she is believed to eat human flesh, shows that she has ceased to be a normal human being. If anybody ill-treats a witch, she would not have sympathizers, even among her own children. Those who sympathize with a witch may also be accused of witchcraft. Most people refrain from defending a person who would have been accused of practicing witchcraft. Some abusive men, can easily take advantage of that by accusing their wives of witchcraft in order to deprive them of the community's empathy. A witch can be beaten up, divorced, or even exiled, and no one is supposed to empathize with her. Some Shona people would say, "*Regai arobwe, muroyi*," which can be translated as, "Let her be beaten, for she is a witch." According to Abraham Akrong, witchcraft accusations of women can lead to their marginalization by making them social outcasts.[23] The accusations may isolate them from their community and relatives. That isolation may render them vulnerable to abuse from family members and other villagers.

For some people, claiming to be a witch is a way of gaining power, and threatening their enemies in the society. It is true that some people lack economic, political, and physical power, yet they need them for survival. Some weak people are not respected and recognized in the communities in which they live. Ordinarily, some people try to compensate for that lack

---

22. Ibid., 140.
23. Akrong. "A Phenomenology of Witchcraft in Ghana," 53–66.

of power by claiming to be witches. That confession directs the societal attention towards them. People begin to notice them, and talk about them. Some people begin to fear them. Some self-proclaimed witches end up getting favors that they would not have got if they had not confessed to be witches. Their children also share the power that their parents are given by the community. They are not molested or bullied at school, for both teachers and other students fear the witches' retaliation. The witches' crops are not destroyed by other villagers' stray livestock, for the cow herders take extra care not to offend the witches. Thieves may stop attempting to steal from a witch because the witch might apprehend them using *rukwa*.

These scholars have also argued that we may not rely on the testimony that is extracted from people using torture. Among the Shona, some witchcraft confessions were extracted through compulsion, particularly during child labor. This confession is known as *kudura*. The Shona suspected that any protracted and difficult labor was a result of some sexual or social misdemeanor that would have been committed by the woman. Two offenses were usually suspected—infidelity and witchcraft. The midwives always encouraged women in that predicament to confess their offences to facilitate the safe birthing of the babies. Some women would confess without being forced by anyone because of the labor pangs. Others would be compelled to confess using torture. Sometimes a metal object would be placed in the fire until it became red hot, and then is used to coerce the birthing woman to confess. Occasionally, some women would confess that they were witches so that they would be spared from the torture. Shona people took those forced confessions seriously, although most of them would have been given as an attempt to escape pain. Most of those confessions were made to the midwives in confidence, who either shared them with the husband, or kept them to themselves.

Christianity and Witchcraft

Most Christian missionaries and European colonizers came to Africa after the European witch hunting in which about 300,000 so-called witches are believed to have perished.[24] Most Europeans knew about the devastating effects of witchcraft beliefs on the powerless members of the society, particularly women and the old. Some of them were genuinely upset to discover that most Africans tenaciously believed that witchcraft was a reality. Some of the early Europeans in Africa witnessed the ostracization, lynching, and

---

24. Parrinder, *Witchcraft*, 35.

shaming of witches by their societal leaders. Some of them wrote home about the horrors of those Africans that were accused of witchcraft.

Some missionaries preached against the belief in witchcraft, and defended the accused witches, to the greatest shock of most Africans. For Africans, practicing witchcraft was against the principles of the Christian message, which encouraged people to live peacefully as brothers and sisters, and shunning all evil doings. The Christian God was a God of justice who would punish the evil doers on the day of judgment. For most Africans, witches were anti-social and evil, and because of that they were supposed to be punished in one way or another. Now, for the missionaries to defend witches was not only a betrayal to the victims of witchcraft, but also a terrible blow to the religious perspectives of the African people.

The missionaries' argument was simple and straightforward—witchcraft did not exist and all beliefs surrounding it were superstitious. They had a different perspective concerning the occurrence of sickness, misfortunes, and death. Some of their explanations of the causes of diseases were equally weird to Africans. They accused tiny creatures such as mosquitoes and houseflies of spreading diseases. For Africans, if it was true that mosquitoes and houseflies spread diseases, why were most of them still alive since these creatures spared no human being and household? As if that was not weird enough, the Europeans accused invisible creatures (germs) of causing diseases, and when Africans asked to see these germs, they were told that they could only be visualized by specialists using powerful microscopes. Africans argued that the same applied to witches: only specialists such as traditional medical practitioners could visualize them using their spiritual microscopes.

The missionaries' demonization of witchcraft beliefs found more substance in the enactment of anti-witchcraft laws in several African countries. These laws were almost similar in the sense that they intended to punish the people who accused others of witchcraft, those who claimed to have knowledge of witchcraft, particularly, traditional medical practitioners, and those who received money in connection with the identification of witches. In Zimbabwe, the Witchcraft Suppression Act (Chapter 73) was promulgated in 1899, on August 18. This law frustrated many Africans because it was intended to let the evil person—the witch go Scot free, yet punishing the life-saver—the traditional medical practitioner. The missionaries' position on witchcraft was vindicated. Anyone who accused another person of witchcraft would be dealt with severely by the law. Unfortunately, the law did not eradicate the witchcraft beliefs from the indigenous people's mentality. It also failed to deter the traditional medical practitioners from doing their job of identifying witches and healing the victims. However, they had to change their tactics to escape the wrath of the law. Most of them stopped naming the witches when they were consulted by the families of the sick persons. Some would point out that the misfortune, sickness or death was a result of witchcraft, and they would ask leading questions so that the relatives of the victim would identify the witch who was responsible. This way of identifying a witch was not as reliable as the traditional way of doing it.

Some African Christians took advantage of this bitterness and frustration by starting their own churches that are popularly known as African Independent Churches. These churches were founded by Africans for Africans for the purpose of preaching a contextualized and inculturated gospel to them. Many reasons have been put forward for the mushrooming of African Independent Churches, but the issue of witchcraft was one of the most crucial ones. The pastors in these churches preached that witchcraft was a reality that needed the church's attention. They claimed to have the power to exorcize witches of their witchcraft and to heal the victims. Some of them prophesied about the future, and could forewarn their followers of the possible attacks by witches.

African Independent Churches have become ubiquitous in Africa. In Zimbabwe, they are popularly known as *Mapositori, Mazioni, and Mapentecosta, or Chechi Dzemweya)*. In their liturgy, there is a stage when the *prophets* foretell the future of some of their members, and diagnose the causes of sickness of the sick members. For them, witchcraft is one of the most popular cause. They also perform faith-healing of the sick. They cleanse members who would have been victimized by evil spirits *(mamhepo* or *mweya yesvina)*. Some of these churches have been criticized for distracting their followers from seeking Western medical attention earlier, which is believed to be more effective.

It should be noted that most of the Shona people who have remained members of the mainlines churches such as the Roman Catholic Church, Reformed Church of Zimbabwe, Anglican, United Methodist Church, and many others, continue to believe in witchcraft. Some members of such churches clandestinely visit traditional medical practitioners and African Independent Churches' prophets whenever they encounter a misfortune such as sickness, death, accident, and bad luck *(munyama)*. Some have a dual religious allegiance, for they are mainstream Christians by the day, and Shona traditionalists by the night.

Witchcraft is one of the Shona beliefs that Christianity has failed to eradicate. Many Shona people would pretend that they no longer believe in witchcraft when their health and fortunes are perfect. But most of them quickly seek traditional medical practitioners' and prophets' expertise when they encounter sicknesses and misfortunes that cannot be explained by natural causes. When Western medicines do not seem to yield expected results, some Shona patients switch to the traditional medicines. Mutual witchcraft accusations are still very common among the Shona.

Perhaps Aylward Shorter's advice makes a lot of sense, at this point. He thinks that it is a waste of time to argue for or against the existence of witchcraft. The belief is indelibly ingrained in the blood of most Africans. They are not willing to let go the belief because of the vacuum that would be left if they do. For him, the "people's interest must be diverted from the morbid preoccupation with witches."[25] He suggests the introduction of demonology. This diversion has already happened among the Pentecostal and Evangelical Christians in Africa, who talk of the devil and demons as if they were physical beings. However, that diversion has not produced the desired results because Africans still believe that the devil and witches influence each other, and the terms are sometimes used interchangeably. Perhaps the perpetuity of the African's belief in witchcraft proves that witchcraft exists, or that no foreign religious belief can easily replace it.

---

25. Shorter, *African Culture and the Christian Church*, 144.

7

Alien Spirits

The spirits that are disallowed to become ancestors are not permanently banished from the Shona society—they still linger around. Although they are forbidden from coming back into their families of origins as ancestors, they are free to look for other families that might accept them as alien spirits. These spirits bear no grudge against their relatives, for they understand why they cannot return to their families of origin as ancestors. They know that they do not qualify to become ancestors, for they were never married, and did not beget children. For the traditional Shona, every person who has reached the marriageable age must get married, and every marriage is expected to be blessed with children. Unfortunately, death does not discriminate against unmarried people; it also consumes them, which is almost disastrous to the future of their spirits, for they are automatically disqualified from joining their dead relatives as ancestors.

The spirits of those who die before marriage and have no children are told not to come back as ancestors because they have not left children who might need their protection. Children are responsible for performing the cleansing ceremony (*kurova guva*) that initiates the spirit of the dead into ancestorhood. After death, the spirit of the unfortunate youth is believed to wander about in search of a host who might accept him as a friendly alien spirit (*shavi*). A *shavi* is a spirit of a person that does not qualify to become an ancestor, which searches for a host among strangers, and upon being accepted, imparts certain talents and skills on that host.

Categories of Alien Spirits (*Mashavi*)

Social Alien Spirits

Basically, there are four categories of *shavi* spirits among the Shona. The first type comprises the social spirits. These spirits bestow special talents and gifts upon their hosts. Soon after death, the spirits of young people wander among the strangers in search of recognition and acceptance. The nerve-racking and tedious search for a willing host is believed to take a long time. Occasionally, some impatient spirits may impose themselves upon unwilling hosts. Once the *shavi* identifies a host, it makes her sick from an inexplicable disease. The relatives of that host may consult a traditional medical practitioner, who is likely to enlighten them about the cause of the sickness. Usually the would-be host must accept the spirit for her to recuperate from her mysterious illness. If the chosen person does not want to accept the *shavi* spirit, she and her family may seek the help of a healer who can cast out the spirit, and prevents it from bothering her. However, in the past, many chosen hosts would accept the spirit once they were assured of its identity, character, and talents. Many Shona people were almost always willing to accept the spirit for they knew that most social alien spirits could impart divination and healing skills on their hosts. Consequently, the acceptance of alien spirits could immensely enrich the host. In repayment to the spirit, the host must appease the spirit with libation, food, clothes, blankets, animal blood, weapons, and ornaments such as beads.[1]

The acceptance ritual is performed under the guidance of a sponsor, usually a senior traditional medical practitioner. The ritual involves the brewing of beer and buying of the spiritual garb depending on the type of the *shavi*. The acceptance ritual starts on the eve of the day of the ritual, and ends at the end of the next day. All other hosts of alien spirits (*mashavi*) who live in the neighborhood gather at the home of the host, and dance with her throughout the ceremony. This dancing encourages the *shavi* to manifest itself by openly possessing the host. Ordinarily, the *shavi* gets possession of the host during the ritual dances, and is offered its official regalia. From that day on, the *shavi* is officially recognized by the family of the host as one of the spiritual members of that family. Once the *shavi* has been accepted, and publicly possesses the host, it may also invite other *shavi* spirits that have different talents to come to the same host. It is common for a person to host several alien spirits, each of them possessing a particular skill. My grandmother's sister, Mai Zhezha, was a host to six different healing *mashavi*, each with a particular expertise. Matengarufu was summoned to perform divination and exorcisms of *ngozi* and evil spirits (*mamhepo*). Chipunha was a specialist in children's ailments. VaMuchembere specialized in midwifery, pediatrics, and adult sicknesses. Zinyama was specialized in treating illnesses caused by *zvitsinga/muposo* (trap/landmine witchcraft). Zinyama was also specialized in the sucking out (*kuruma*) method of healing, in which harmful objects, which are maliciously placed in the victim's body by the witches, are removed. Masvosvera and Sekanomusi were general practitioners and entertainers.

1. Rayner, *The Tribe and Its Successors*, 101.

Sometimes the *shavi* approaches the would-be host in dreams as a manifestation of its request. The chosen person may dream of herbs, dancing, and singing *shavi* music. Among some Karanga groups, it is also believed that if one sees or dreams of a python, it is a sign that some *shavi* wants to possess her. If the dream is recurrent, her family may consult a traditional medical practitioner who affirms the presence of the *shavi*, and may prescribe the rituals to be performed as a sign of acceptance of the spirit.

Sometimes the *shavi* refuses to openly possess the host during the acceptance ritual. In cases like that, another acceptance ritual must be performed until the host gets possessed. If the *shavi* never possesses the host openly that could be interpreted as a sign that the consulted medical practitioner was mistaken.

Social Alien Spirits

There are many sub-types of social alien spirits. *Majukwa* are believed to emanate from God, and can only possess the sons of Mwari.[2] The sons of Mwari were the men who were dedicated to the service of the Shona God of Matonjeni. The *Majukwa* color is black. *Majukwa* are believed to be responsible for rainmaking. Their mediums were the messengers that the Shona communities would send to Matonjeni to ask for rain. They also officiate at the rainmaking ritual (*mutoro/mukwerere*). Their songs are associated with rainmaking. One of the most popular of such songs goes as follows:

> *Warivona dziva remvura, iyooo*
> (You have seen the pool of water).
>
> *Wairivona dziva remvura, Zame*
> (You have seen the pool of water at Zame).
>
> *Matonjeni kunotsva moto, iyoooo*
> (Fire is burning at Matonjeni).
>
> *Warivona dzivaremvura Zame*
> (You have seen the pool of water at Zame).

Chipunha shavi is believed to be fond of possessing young girls who would be playful under the possession by the *shavi*. They may climb up trees and talk in strange tongues.[3] *Chipunha* also can heal. *Madlozi* is a type of *mashavi* that is believed to have their origin among the Ndebele

---

2. Bullock, *The Mashona*, 148.
3. Rayner, *The Tribe and Its Successors*, 147.

people, who after being rejected by their relatives, come to possess the Shona people. Such spirits impart the art of dancing, healing, and fighting on their hosts. Women who are hosts to such spirits are known for their boxing skills. *Madlozi* favor red and white colors. The ritual songs are sung in Ndebele, and the hosts speak in Ndebele when possessed. They are also healers. *Muzungu shavi* type comes from the either the Portuguese or English settlers who would have died in Zimbabwe. When the host is possessed, she speaks in Portuguese or English. She may ask for European food such as rice, tea, bread, and so on. The host may be a healer, and may sing some English songs when possessed. *Muzungu shavi* may ask for special attire and is usually very smart.[4]

The names given to social *mashavi* depend on the origin of the spirit. *Madzviti shavi* originates from the Ndebele. *Changani shavi* originates from the Shangani people, and so on. Michael Gelfand has a detailed explanation of the characteristics of several *shavi* spirits.[5]

Anti-Social Alien Spirits

The anti-social *mashavi* are evil because they tend to impose their anti-social behavior and talents on their hosts. The anti-social *mashavi* are spirits of the people who would have been evil during their earthly lives. Some of these spirits would have been rejected or exorcized by their family members. The search for a host by anti-social spirits resembles that of good spirits except that anti-social spirits do not wait to be accepted by the hosts. Most of them forcefully take possession of the unwilling, and sometimes unaware hosts, and begin to use them to pursue their nefarious missions.

The most notorious of anti-social *mashavi* is the *mamutsamurimo*, which can be translated as, the revival of the trade. *Mamutsa* comes from the Shona verb *kumutsa*, which means to awaken someone or revive something. *Murimo* is a noun, which comes from the verb *kurima*, which means to farm. This *shavi* may be a spirit of a relative who was a witch, particularly a grandmother, who comes back to use another family member as a witch. The bewitching spirit comes back to revive the witchcraft trade in the family, which would have expired with the witch's death. Such people would have been banished from their homes before they died, or would have been denied themselves the opportunity of becoming ancestors because of their anti-social behavior. Both strange and family spirits can become *mamutsamurimo*.

4. Gelfand, *Shona Ritual, with Reference to the Chaminuka Cult*, 137.
5. Read Gelfand, *Shona Ritual, with Reference to the Chaminuka Cult*, 121–52.

In most cases, the host does not know that she is used by a bewitching spirit (*mamutsamurimo*) until she is identified by other people as a witch. It is also believed that the host may suspect being used by such a spirit by analyzing her dreams in which she bewitches people. Most targeted hosts do not accept the *mamutsamurimo,* but they find themselves trapped. Efforts to exorcize *mamutsamurimo* may be futile since such spirits are stubborn and would resist any attempt to exorcize them. But some traditional medical practitioners claim that they can cast out such spirits. The casting out rituals are normally performed at crossroads to ensure that the spirit takes possession of the first person to pass through that road, lest it comes back to its former host.

At times, such spirits are symbolically placed on a live black goat or chicken, which is then driven into the bush. Anybody who comes across such a goat or chicken and slaughters it, becomes the new host of the spirit. If the bewitching spirit refuses to be cast out, some families do perform rituals to appease it so that it remains dormant. Those rituals can be categorized as *bira reChivanhu/Chikaranga* (traditional beer ritual), without specifying its purpose. The rituals are performed early in the morning before the arrival of the invited guests. The appeased spirits are believed to waylay those who arrive early for the ritual beer, and may possess them.

In the traditional Shona society, some people accepted such spirits, and began to ply their trade of witchcraft. Such willing hosts of *mamutsamurimo* would then appease such spirits through their cannibalistic rituals. The Shona believe that such spirits do not just choose their hosts randomly, but they look for people who possess anti-social traits such as selfishness (*kunyima*), sulkiness (*kusindimara*), and individualism (*undingoveni*). Any person of such a character is suspected of being a witch, even if she is not.

Another anti-social *shavi* is called *chisinha*, and it can possess both men and women. *Chisinha* is the spirit of a person who would have died before marriage, and is angry for dying before tying the knot, and begetting children. *Chisinha* wanders about in search of a host of the opposite sex, and when it finds him, it considers him its husband. If the *chisinha* is the spirit of a man, it may consider itself the secret husband of the host. Usually, *chisinha* chooses an unmarried host, and prevents her from getting married. Some of the *zvisinha* allow the host to get a boyfriend, but may not permit her to be intimate with him. Whenever the two try to be intimate, the host gets possessed by the *chisinha*, and may assault the boyfriend. If a person who has reached marriageable age fails to get a marriage partner, the Shona are likely to suspect the presence of *chisinha*. Some traditional medical practitioners claim to have the power to exorcize such spirits. My grandmother's sister, Mai Zhezha, had a place (*Dambiro raMai Zhezha*) at the foot of Chitakai

Mountain, where she performed such rituals. It is believed that once the ritual is performed, the affected man or woman can get married.

The other undesirable *shavi* is one that causes the host to have an uncontrollable and insatiable sexual desire (*shavi revarume/vakadzi*). Some of the chosen hosts are believed to end up as prostitutes because they cannot hold a marriage for a long time. The *shavi* can possess both women and men. However, most unfaithful men can get away with it because the Shona culture permits them to marry as many wives as they wish. Moreover, Shona men's infidelity does not raise the same condemnation as that of women. Some women who claim to have that *shavi* say that whenever it gets possession of them, they end up getting involved in illicit love affairs without planning for it. Families that realize that one of their daughters has such a *shavi*, may consult a traditional medical practitioner, who is likely to advise them to perform a ritual with the intention of exorcising such a spirit. In most cases, this *shavi* does not publicly and openly possess its host.

The thieving *shavi (roumbavha)* is detested by most Shona people. Again, this *shavi* is inherent, and its host suffers from an uncontrollable and irresistible desire to steal. It is believed that if the host of such an alien spirit fails to steal anything for a long period, he may become sick. Such a host is believed to perform a ritual in which he stages the stealing of one of his items, just to appease the *shavi*. The stealing may start when the host is still young, and may continue despite the discipline of the host by his parents and the law enforcement agents. Some Shona people think that this *shavi* assists the host in identifying objects to steal, and makes their owners easy targets. If the thief (*mbavha*) comes at night, his thieving spirit makes the victim to sleep soundly only to wake up when the thief is gone.

Inherent Alien Spirits

The third category of alien spirits comprises inherent *mashavi* that never openly possess their hosts. Their presence is sometimes sensed through the skills or talents that a person has in doing something. One of these *mashavi* is called *jeranyama,* and it is a hunting *shavi*. It is believed that the host dreams of where he can get the game and when. Usually, the wife or mother of such a hunter performs rituals after the person would have brought home game meat. One of the rituals is to give the hunter roasted groundnuts, which are believed to be the favorite snack of the *jeranyama*. The hunter may have taboos that he upholds as dictated by the *shavi*.

There are many other *mashavi* that fall in this category, such as *shavi rekurima* (farming spirit), *shavi rekumanya* (running spirit), *shavi rekugona* (spirit of intelligence), and many others. Some scholars have dismissed these *mashavi* as mere explanations that the Shona gave to inborn gifts and talents that people have.[6] To some extent, Rayner's theory makes sense because most people who are believed to have *mashavi* are skilled in one way or the other. However, the Shona feel that some people are so talented that something from outside of them must explain such talents.

Animal and Object Alien Spirits

The last category of alien spirits consists of spirits of animals and objects that possess human beings as *mashavi*. The most popular of these *mashavi* is the *shavi regudo* (baboon spirit). The host of that *shavi* behaves like a baboon when he is possessed by it. The host makes the baboon sounds, scratches her body, and may climb up trees. This *shavi* has no special talent except entertaining people because its host is a good dancer. This phenomenon has led some outsiders to postulate that the Shona believe that all things have spirits. It is difficult to tell why the Shona think that the baboon, of all the animals, has a spirit that can possess human beings. There has been mention of the *ndege* (aeroplane) *shavi*, which is another phenomenon that suggests a belief in animism among the Shona. However, it is difficult to verify the authenticity of baboon and aeroplane alien spirits. Most scholars doubt their authenticity.

Alien Spirits and Christianity

Mashavi suffered a great blow because of the acceptance of Christianity by the Shona people. Just like they did to ancestor veneration, the missionaries vehemently condemned alien spirits. They attacked the traditional medical practitioners who used these spirits in their healing and divination practices. When the Witchcraft Suppression Act was promulgated in 1899, it became a pernicious offence to claim to have the knowledge of witchcraft, and that left the traditional medical practitioners without jobs. Although they could still perform their healing practices, they were not allowed to diagnose the causes of the ailment.

The introduction of hospitals and Western medicines also dealt them a serious blow. They had to compete for patients with Western physicians, who were assisted by missionaries and their surrogates in belittling the traditional healing practices. Sooner the Shona discovered that in most

---

6. Rayner, *The Tribe and Its Successors*, 100.

cases, the Western medical methods were quicker and more efficacious than their methods, and they then embraced them. For instance, Western doctors could operate on a pregnant woman to save both the baby and mother, which African midwives could not do. Westerners could easily and effectively repair broken bones. The Shona people who continued to visit traditional medical practitioners would do that as a last resort, usually after trying the Western medicines.

During the Liberation Struggle for the independence of Zimbabwe (1976-80), the freedom fighters under Mr. Robert Mugabe revived and popularized ancestral veneration by affirming the ancestors' involvement in the war. They also banned the worship of God in the areas where they operated. However, the belief in *mashavi,* and their healing activities were not revived because the freedom fighters relied on Western medicines to treat their ailments. Occasionally, they consulted traditional medical practitioners in their witch hunting endeavor that resulted in many innocent people losing their lives. Some traditional medical practitioners became very unpopular because of such wanton killings of the people who were accused of witchcraft. At independence, in 1980, some Shona people gradually abandoned ancestral veneration, and went back to their Christian churches.

When some hosts of *mashavi* were tired of their condemnation by the missionaries, they converted to African Independent Churches, where they assumed a new role as *prophets.* In some African Independent Churches, they continue to perform divination and healing, but in a manner, that is compatible with the teachings of the churches in which they are members. They are still the same traditional medical practitioners. What has only changed is the context of their healing activities. They still treat people who suffer from the same old traditional symptoms. What is interesting about them is that some of them condemn *mashavi* as evil. This switching to Christianity has saved *mashavi* and the traditional healing methods from dying out completely. The Shona now get most of the traditional medical practitioners' services from the African Independent Churches' prophets. Unlike ancestor veneration, the *mashavi* veneration is almost dead among the Shona of Zimbabwe.

8

Traditional Medical Practitioners

One of the research challenges that the early Western writers and researchers of African Traditional Religion encountered was the lack of the appropriate and respectful terminology for some of the phenomena that they observed. Consequently, some of them ended up using derogatory and unacceptable terminology such as savage, native, tribe, paganism, animism, totemism, heathenism, and others, about Africans and their religions.[1] There are primarily three factors that might have led to the use of these pejorative and misleading terms.

First, most early Western writers spoke the English language, and might have had problems in finding the English equivalency of some African terms. In Africa, they experienced and observed some phenomena that they had never seen before, and for which they had no appropriate equivalents. Likewise, they also had European terms and ideas that they wanted to introduce to Africans, but since those were not part of the African experience, they could not find appropriate terms to use. Some of the African translators that they sometimes employed were limited in their understanding of the English language, and could not help them very much. Some writers ended up using whatever word they thought would make sense to their European audience, for whom the research and writings were undertaken.

Second, these writers had a different worldview from that of Africans, and that led to their limitations in understanding and interpreting the phenomena that they observed in Africa. A worldview is an inherited and acquired framework through which people understand and interpret their experiences. A child is born within a worldview, but without a worldview of its own. What becomes its worldview is imparted unto it by the significant others, friends, teachers, and its environment. A worldview includes, but is not limited to religion, food, music, language, clothes, dance, and relationships. Ordinarily, most people think that their way of doing things, and understanding the phenomena are perfect and superior to other people's ways. Many people remain entrapped in such a limiting and prejudicial

---

1. For a detailed exploration of those terms read, Idowu, *African Traditional Religion*, 109–36. A Synthesis of those terms can also be read in Chitakure, *The Pursuit of the Sacred*, 53–58.

mentality unless they begin to explore other cultures, peoples, and worldviews, open-mindedly. An objective approach to other people's culture enables the researcher to appreciate some of the new cultural experiences that seem strange and weird at first, but become normal as one continues to experience and reflect on them. To read about other people's culture is rewarding, but might not be as beneficial as experiencing that same culture. Moreover, there is more to culture than a people's language. Some of the Westerners who had mastered the indigenous languages of Africa remained prisoners of their worldviews that prevented them from appreciating some of the African cultures.

Third, because of the cultural and religious superiority that were part of their worldviews, some of the Western writers deliberately decided to use terms that would suggest and promote the inferiority of Africans and their religions when compared to the European culture and Christianity. Those writers were not fools, for they were marketing experts, selling a religion to a people that already had its own religion. They were men on a mission to bring Christianity, commerce, and *civilization* to Africa, and had to confirm the non-existence of such ideologies in Africa, prior to their arrival. Of course, most of them sincerely believed that the European civilization, culture, and religion were superior to any other, and that Africans needed a new religion, culture, and *civilization*, if they were to be saved from their backwardness.

Witchdoctor or Medical Practitioner?

Some of the terms that were used reflect the writers or researchers' derision of Africans and their religious traditions. One of the phenomena that faced such unwarranted bias was the African traditional healer, whom I shall call, the traditional medical practitioner henceforth. The early and later Western writers referred to him as the *witch-doctor*. It is inconceivable to imagine how and why such a noble profession ended up having that degrading and confusing nomenclature. Geoffrey Parrinder aptly describes the confusion when he writes, "No name has suffered more distortion and misunderstanding than that of the witch-doctor. To many people the witch-doctor is the chief witch, the devil of the magical art."[2] What is surprising is that Parrinder went ahead and used the same term that he confessed to be misleading.

The name *witch-doctor* is a combination of two diametrically contradictory terms—*witch* and *doctor*. The Western writers exactly knew the

2. Parrinder, *Witchcraft*, 181.

meanings of both words. They knew that a witch, whether imagined or real, was an evil person, who utilized clandestine and mysterious powers to harm others. On the other hand, a doctor was a healer, a bringer of life, whose desire was to save life by preventing people from contracting diseases, diagnosing the causes of sickness, and curing those who became sick. It is mind-boggling to see such incompatible terms being combined to refer to the African traditional doctor. There were reasons for using that term. It could be that these writers had been informed that the traditional medical practitioner could do either harm or good with his powers and medicines, depending on what he intended to do at that given time. Consequently, he can be referred to as a *witch*, since he had the knowledge of harmful medicines and procedures. He was also a *doctor* because he had the knowledge of medicines and procedures that could save lives. It seems that the writers lacked empathetic logic because the European doctor did the same. He had the knowledge of both harmful and life-saving medicines and procedures, yet they did not refer to him as a *witch-doctor*.

It has also been argued that the writers used that nomenclature to make it clear that the traditional medical practitioner concerned himself more with effects and ailments caused by witchcraft. To a certain extent, it is true that most of his patients were victims of witchcraft. But, there was more to it than that. Some traditional medical practitioners also helped women to give birth. Some presided over marriages. They also treated people who were injured by wild animals, and those bitten by snakes. Some were ritual practitioners who initiated boys and girls into adulthood. They also presided over ancestral and rainmaking rituals. Some of them were counselors and psychologists. Even if one buys the argument that the traditional medical practitioner concerned himself more with effects of witchcraft than other spheres of health, it would still be unjustified to call him a *witch-doctor*. Moreover, traditional medical practitioners' sphere of influence went beyond treating sicknesses caused by witchcraft.

It seems that the name witch-doctor was coined to differentiate an African doctor from a European doctor. For some of the early European writers and missionaries, an African had to be a *witch* to be a doctor. He had to be both evil and good at the same time. To call him a doctor would be tantamount to bringing him up to the position of the European doctor. The name *witch-doctor* was intended to justify legislating against him by some colonial governments.[3] The truth of the matter was that the so-called *witch-doctor* was a medical practitioner in his own right. Up to the period of the coming of the Europeans to Africa, he had managed to render his services

---

3. Parrinder, *Witches*, 181.

to his people fruitfully. Like what happened to the European physician's patients, some of the African traditional medical practitioner's patients died, but the rest survived.

David Livingstone (1813–73) who was a missionary, medical doctor, and explorer in Africa, had a wonderful conversation with the rain doctor among the Bakuena (VaKwena) of King Sechele of Botswana. At the time of the conversation, Livingstone had managed to convert the indigenous people to Christianity, but the new coverts had become anxious when a drought came. They prayed to the Christian God, and the new God seemed to be indifferent to their need of rain. They persuaded David Livingstone to allow them to perform their traditional rainmaking rituals, and it seems that the missionary, who was skeptical of their rituals, was reluctant to give them the permission to induce the rain. Livingstone told them to abandon their traditional medicines and rituals, and then give all their trust to the Christian God. The rain doctor responded by saying that God had told Africans a different story, and that their ways and medicines were as good as European ways and medicines. The following is an excerpt from the conversation:

> **Rain Doctor (R. D.)** . . . He has given us the knowledge of certain medicines by which we can make rain. WE do not despise those things which you possess, though we are ignorant of them. We don't understand your book, yet we don't despise it. YOU ought not to despise our little knowledge, though you are ignorant of it.
>
> **Medical Doctor (M. D.)** I don't despise what I am ignorant of; I only think you are mistaken in saying that you have medicines which can influence the rain at all.
>
> **R. D.** That's just the way people speak when they talk on a subject of which they have no knowledge. When we first opened our eyes, we found our forefathers making rain, and we follow in their footsteps. You, who send to Kuruman for corn, and irrigate your garden, may do without rain; WE cannot manage in that way. If we had no rain, the cattle would have no pasture, the cows give no milk, our children become lean and die, our wives run away to other tribes who do make rain and have corn, and the whole tribe become dispersed and lost; our fire would go out.
>
> **M. D.** I quite agree with you as to the value of the rain; but you cannot charm the clouds by medicines. You wait till you see the clouds come, then you use your medicines, and take the credit which belongs to God only.

R. D. I use my medicines, and you employ yours; we are both doctors, and doctors are not deceivers. You give a patient medicine. Sometimes God is pleased to heal him by means of your medicine; sometimes not—he dies. When he is cured, you take the credit of what God does. I do the same. Sometimes God grants us rain, sometimes not. When he does, we take the credit of the charm. When a patient dies, you don't give up trust in your medicine, neither do I when rain fails. If you wish me to leave off my medicines, why continue your own?[4]

To call a traditional medical practitioner a *witch-doctor* was not only slanderous to an individual medical practitioner, but also to the whole traditional medical profession. These people were medical practitioners in their own right. Therefore, I will refer to him as the traditional medical practitioner (*n'anga/chiremba*). It should be noted that, unlike in other parts of Africa, among the Shona of Zimbabwe, there were/are male and female traditional medical practitioners.[5] The pronoun *he* is used for convenience's sake, and without any prejudice intended.

The Calling

How does one become a traditional medical practitioner? In the past, there were many ways in which one was called to the traditional medical field. Some people discovered their calls through dreams in which they dreamt of herbs and methods of healing people.[6] It was believed that those dreams came from the healer spirits that wanted to pass on their skills to the person who dreamt about healing. Some people would clearly remember the herbs that they would have been shown in their dreams. Some of those spirits would be family spirits of the dreaming person. But other spirits would be alien spirits seeking recognition and acceptance, for which they rewarded the host by the impartation of healing expertise.

Among some Karanga groups, it was believed that if someone dreamt of a python, it meant that there was some healer alien spirit that wanted to impart healing skills on him. Usually the person who would have had such a dream would consult a traditional medical practitioner for advice on what to do next. Most of the time, he would be asked to perform a ritual at which the spirit was summoned through drumming and dancing. Once the spirit announced its presence by publicly possessing the host, then he could

---

4. David Livingstone, *Missionary Travels and Researches in South Africa*, chapter 1.
5. Evans-Pritchard, *Witchcraft, Oracles, and Magic among the Azande*, 72.
6. Bourdillon, *The Shona Peoples*, 165.

start performing as a medical practitioner. Such a healer would sometimes get possessed by the healer spirit, and would go into the bush to gather the needed medicinal herbs. However, most healers would remember the herbs that they would have dreamt about, and did not need any spiritual possession to retrieve them. Some *n'angas* were possessed by several healer spirits, each with its own specialty. The host would listen to the sick person's history, and would then summon the relevant healing spirit.

Some traditional medical practitioners had a dramatic calling. It is believed that some would be victims of a kidnaping by a mermaid (*njuzu*). These people would have been snatched by the *njuzu*, and would disappear into the pool of water for months or even years. It is believed that during that period, the captured person would be coached by the mermaid spirit on how to heal people. When they finally emerged from the pool, they would bring their medicines and other healing paraphernalia that are needed in their profession. The mermaid would only release the captured person after the performance of an appeasement ritual by the victim's relatives.

Some traditional medical practitioners' calling was not so easy. The one being called would become sick, and his family would consult a medical practitioner, who would tell them the cause of his sickness. Usually, they were told to perform a *shavi* welcoming ritual that involved beer drinking, dancing, and singing. Some people would become possessed by the healer spirit during that ritual. It was believed that once the ritual was performed, the sick person would recuperate, and would begin to heal people using the skills that would have been given to him by the spirit. Sometimes the intended host would suffer from barrenness, and upon consulting a traditional medical practitioner, her family would be told to perform a ritual, at which she had to accept the healer spirit.

Some people underwent training in medicine and related issues before they could operate as healers. There were people who would attach themselves to a traditional medical practitioner as an assistant for a long period. Most of these people would have no intention of becoming *n'angas* themselves, but their closeness and interaction with a professional traditional medical practitioner would enable them to acquire some of his skills. Most *n'angas* needed assistants to help them with the digging and crushing of herbs. In the process of rendering such help, most of the lay assistants would acquire the knowledge of the use of some curative herbs. Some of those assistants were translators of the *n'angas*, and again would acquire the knowledge and skills of divination and healing. Most of the time this discipleship was offered to a relative of the *n'anga* for free. If the assistant was a stranger, who would have come in search of training, then he had to pay fees to the *n'anga*. In most cases of this nature, the *n'anga* could only pass on the knowledge of herbs and how to use them, but not the healing spirits.

There were some traditional medical practitioners who were not healers in the strict sense of the word, but had immense knowledge of herbs. For instance, most midwives were not *n'angas* in the strict sense of the word, but they had the knowledge of the procedures and medicines that were needed to facilitate or induce the safe birth of a baby. They too had the knowledge of medicines that were used to immunize the baby from both physical and spiritual ailments. Some of them knew how to predetermine the gender of the child, which was known as *kushandura nyoka*. They too had the expertise to cure barrenness (*kusimikira*). The Shona word *kusimikira* is an extension of the verb, *kusima*, which means to plant. When the word is used in connection to barrenness, it means to induce pregnancy using medicines.

Those sacred practitioners who performed circumcision of the boys had the expertise in performing surgical procedures, and treating complicated cases of infection. The Shona also had people who specialized in medicines that enhanced sexual virility. All these people would have learnt their trade from the elders, spirits, and *n'angas*. Some of them were not *n'angas* per se, but they performed duties of medical practitioners.

Types of Traditional Medical Practitioners

Although there are several types of traditional medical practitioners such as diviners, midwives, and herbalists, spirit mediums are the most important. Most powerful diviners are believed to be aided by spirits, and they use both the spirits and medical dices called *hakata* to diagnose the cases that are brought to them.[7] The *hakata* can be made from half shells of a certain tree, flat bones, or curved wood. During divination, these are thrown to the ground by both the enquirer and the *n'anga*. Usually the diviner puts a question to the dice before throwing them to the ground, and then infer the answer from the position in which they land on the ground.[8] It is the diviner's responsibility to interpret the dices contextually. The same dice and position can mean different things to different enquirers.

Those who need the service of a diviner usually visit one that is reputable for his ability (*kuvona*), and who lives far away from the village of the enquirers. This long-distance consultation is intended to prevent the *n'anga* from using the prior knowledge of his clients that he might have. The *n'anga*

---

7. For an in-depth exploration of *hakata*, read Bourdillon, *The Shona Peoples*, 152–58, and Gelfand, *Shona Religion with Special Reference to the Makorekore*, 108–17.

8. Hubert Bucher, *Spirits and Power*, 116.

should be able to greet his visitors by names and totems, explain the nature of their relationship, and pinpoint the purpose of their visit. It is believed that all this information is given to the diviner in a dream or vision before the arrival of the visitors. Once the *n'anga* manages to do this successfully, then he gains the confidence and trust of the clients. Diviners diagnose the ailment, identify the cause of the problem, and prescribe the appropriate remedy. If a diviner is unable to remedy the situation, he may refer the clients to another diviner. Some diviners do not accept payment (*madza*) until after the recuperation of the patient, which some people believe to be the hallmark of a confident and competent healer.

There are several health conditions for which diviners are consulted. Serious misfortunes bedeviling the family such as death, bad luck, barrenness, and mental illness, may force the Shona to consult a diviner. Sometimes an individual may consult a *n'anga* alone, but it is highly encouraged that all the family members be involved, if they are dealing with a serious problem such as illness or death. Usually, the leader of the family or the affected individual invites other members to consult a diviner together. According to Michael Gelfand, "a mysterious or suspicious event such as the appearance of a snake in the village," would cause a family to consult a diviner.[9] A snake such as *ndara/munzamusha,* or the hooting of owls while sitting on the roof of someone's house would necessitate the consultation of a diviner.

Herbalists may be divided into two categories. The first group comprises those herbalists who only have the expertise of therapeutic herbs, and do not host any healing spirit. These herbalists treat all sorts of ailments, ranging from the common cold to serious illnesses. Some of them receive patients that are referred to them by other diviners. Sacred practitioners such as midwives may fall into this category. In fact, most Shona elders know a few common herbal treatments for common infections such as colds. For instance, it is common knowledge that *zumbani* (of the species, Lippia Javanica) can be used to treat influenza when taken as tea, chewed raw, or smoked as a cigarette. Most Shona elders know herbs that treat snake bites, although complicated bites may need the attention of reputed herbalists. Although the possession of the knowledge of a few herbal treatments does not make anyone a full-fledged herbalist, people with such knowledge may be referred to as herbalists. Usually they prescribe the herbs for their families and friends without charging them anything. The second category consists of those herbalists who are possessed by healing spirits, which inspire them with the knowledge of herbs. Such *n'angas* may do both diagnosis

---

9. Gelfand, *Shona Religion with Special Reference to the Makorekore,* 109.

and healing. It is common to find a *n'anga* who performs divination, and has the knowledge of curative herbs.

In the past, most families had at least one ancestral spirit medium. When something was not well with any member of the family, such an ancestral host would get possessed by the ancestral spirit, and would warn the family of the possible illness or the impending death of one of the family members. Although the host was not a *n'anga*, she could foresee some impending disasters and would then forewarn the family. Occasionally, the family head would summon the ancestral spirit to consult it on issues of interest. To summon the ancestral spirit, the family head would hand ground tobacco (*fodya yebute*) to the ancestral host, which she would place on either of her shoulders without saying a thing, and within a short period the spirit would possess her. Some ancestors would refer sick family members to a *n'anga*. It should be noted that most ancestral hosts are not *n'angas*, but they can see into the future, and forewarn their living family members of impending dangers.

Recently, the *tsikamutanda* type of traditional medical practitioners have taken some Zimbabwean districts by storm. The word *tsikamutanda* is a compound Shona word from *tsika*, which means *step on something*, and *mutanda*, which means *stick*. Hence, *tsikamutanda* is an imperative or command for someone to step on the stick. This term must have its etiology in one of the divination methods of the *n'angas* of this type, who sometimes tell the people who are being vetted for witchcraft to step on a medicinal stick to prove their innocence. These *n'angas* specialize in witch-hunting, exorcisms of witchcraft spirits, and the destruction of other harmful spirts such as *zvikwambo* (goblins). Unlike other traditional medical practitioners, *tsikamutanda n'angas* visit the people in their communities, and offer or impose their services. There is no need for anybody to be sick, for the *tsikamutandas* to visit a particular community to expose the witches and exorcize them of their witchcraft. Once they get the permission from the village head, they gather all the villagers, and begin the verting process. If someone is found to be a witch, he may pay a fee to the *n'angas* to exorcize him of his witchcraft. Occasionally, they are summoned to a village by one of the villagers who would have known of their activities in another village. It is difficult to pinpoint the origin of these *n'angas* because they are itinerary. There have been reports about these healers getting in trouble with the law enforcement agents for fleecing the villagers, and their use of unorthodoxy ways of exposing witches.

Diagnosis

Once a *n'anga* is consulted, she is likely to identify the cause of the misfortune. It is rare for a *n'anga* to ignore the cause of the misfortune. One of the most frequent causes of misfortunes is the avenging spirit. Usually, the avenging spirits attack the family members of the perpetrator of some injustice, who sometimes have no knowledge of the crime that they are being punished for. Sometimes, the misfortunes caused by avenging spirits begin to happen long after the perpetrator is dead. In cases like that, the only way a family might know of the presence of such a spirit is by consulting traditional medical practitioners. The affected family may consult several traditional medical practitioners to confirm their earlier findings. Most of the *n'angas* may also explain to the clients the rituals to be carried out to appease the avenging spirit. Those *n'angas* who are not well versed in dealing with avenging spirits may refer their clients to other *n'angas*. Some *n'angas* claim to have the ability to exorcize avenging spirits although the most conventional remedy for *ngozi* attacks is for the family of the perpetrator to pay reparations to the relatives of the aggrieved spirit.

The other common cause of illnesses, misfortunes, or even deaths is witchcraft. In the past, most medical practitioners would identify the witch and the reason for his malevolent actions. Nowadays, most *n'angas* do not identify the witch by his name because doing so violates the *Witchcraft Suppression Act*. However, the *n'anga* may indirectly reveal the identity of the witch. Occasionally, the family of the sick person might be advised to perform the *gumbwa*, which refers to a situation where the whole village, led by its village head, goes to consult a *n'anga* together. It is believed that the *n'anga* can separate the witches from innocent villagers. The act of being acquitted of witchcraft by a *n'anga* during *gumbwa* is called *kupembera*. If the people identified as witches want to contest the findings of the *n'anga*, they may ask the group to consult several *n'angas*. If the verdict of the first *n'anga* is confirmed by subsequent *n'angas*, then the villagers may return to their village, and would advise the apprehended witches to reverse the effects of their witchcraft.

Sometimes the family of the sick person may consult a *n'anga* alone, and then performs the *kurova bembera* with the assistance of the village head. All the villagers are gathered at their usual meeting place, where the relative of the sick person and the village head publicly profess their knowledge of the identities of the witches without mentioning their names. Also, they may implore the witches to reverse the effects of their witchcraft. Although the names of the witches are not revealed, the villagers may infer them. It is believed that a reasonable witch is likely to give an antidote to the sick person because of the fear of being shamed. In some instances, the *n'anga* may instruct the family of the sick person to relocate the sick person (*kusengudza*) either temporarily or permanently. Sometimes, the whole family may migrate permanently.

Alien spirits (*mashavi*) are sometimes identified as causes of illnesses. They may cause sickness to attract the attention of the person that they intend to make their host. They make that person sick to compel him to accept them. Alien spirits may resort to this way of finding hosts because they are not wanted by their family members as ancestors. They do not qualify to become ancestors because of one reason or another. Once they are accepted by the intended host through a ritual, they may impart their talents on him. The alien spirits that can readily be accepted are healers because they are expected to bring fortunes to the host. In some cases, the host may use a *n'anga* to expel the alien spirit that seeks recognition.

Associated with the alien spirits, as causes of illnesses, are ancestors. Ancestors cause misfortunes for several reasons. First, they may do that to compel their living relatives to honor them. Usually the consulted *n'anga* identifies the aggrieved ancestor, the ritual that needs to be performed, and how it should be performed. Once the ritual is performed, the misfortune should disappear. There are sacred practitioners who contest the idea that ancestors may cause misfortunes to their living family members. They argue that ancestors can only withdraw their protection, which then allows evil spirits to attack their family members. Among some Karanga groups, an ancestor that would have caused the death of a family member, either actively or by negligence, is said to have spilt the blood (*kutsvusa ropa*), and that ancestor is considered dangerous. Ancestors that are considered dangerous are likely to be exorcized.

Sometimes the cause of the sickness is believed to be the existence of a harmful object (*chinhu*) that the witches would have inserted into the body of the victim. Some people claim to experience the object travelling in their body parts such as legs and arms. Once the *chinhu* is identified, some *n'angas* may use their mouths to suck it out (*kuruma*) through incisions that are made by a razor blade. Some *n'angas* use half tennis balls to suck out the objects. Sometimes, objects such as human hair, spoons, forks, bones, live frogs, and many others, may come out of the ailing organ. These objects are shown to the patient, and are eventually burned by the medical practitioner.

Taboos

N'angas have taboos that they should uphold. They should avoid eating some types of food. For instance, some do not eat *sadza* (thick porridge), which is made from finger millet. Every farming season, some *n'angas* must perform a ritual called *kuruma* before they begin to eat the first fruits of the land. They cook pumpkin vegetables, maize cobs, cane, and other fruits of the land, together with medicines, and then eat them. Once they perform this ritual, which is intended to let the ancestors know that the harvest is ready, they may eat any of those freely without falling sick. Most *n'angas* abstain from goat meat that is not slaughtered properly. When one is slaughtering a goat in the way that is ritually acceptable to ancestors, its throat should be tied (*kusunga*) with a string to prevent what is in its belly from getting in contact with the meat. As soon as the goat is slaughtered, the entrails are immediately separated from the rest of the meat so that the meat may not get contaminated.

Traditional Medical Practitioners and Christianity

The coming of Christianity affected the traditional medical practice in several ways.

The first punch was the demonization that was levelled against the traditional medical practitioners themselves. Instead of calling them medical doctors like their counterparts from Europe, they were called *witch-doctors*. In Africa, to call someone a witch has devastating results on that individual. A witch is the chief of evil, and always uses his destructive forces to bring suffering to other people. The *n'angas'* medicines, which were principally herbs, were demonized as well. They were said to belong to Satan, and therefore, unfit and unclean for Christians. The missionaries failed to give credit to the herbs that had kept the people going for thousands of years before their arrival. The African rituals were also ridiculed by the missionaries.

One of the ridiculed rituals was the rainmaking ceremony, which David Livingstone despised as ineffective and fraudulent. Although he claimed to have the knowledge concerning the inefficacy of the rainmaking ritual of the Bakuena people, David Livingstone failed to see the inefficacy of his own God. The rain doctor, with whom he had a conversation, pointed out for him that he was a hypocrite who forced others to completely rely on his Christian God, yet he himself did not trust the same God. That lack of trust was evidenced by the fact that the missionary would send for food from Kuruman, or would irrigate his garden, instead of waiting for his

God's providence. "We cannot manage in that way. If we had no rain, the cattle would have no pasture, the cows give no milk, our children become lean and die, our wives run away to other tribes who do make rain and have corn, and the whole tribe become dispersed and lost; our fire would go out,"[10] explained the rain doctor. Africans fully trusted their medicines, just like the Europeans trusted their own, but to argue that only African medicines were ineffective was hypocritical. These insults did not end with David Livingstone, but were perpetuated by almost every early missionary that came to Africa. Converted Africans were also used to attack African culture, religion, and medicines. This conversion of some Africans caused much division in African families.

The establishment of hospitals in Africa brought about many benefits to the African peoples. The modern medicines were more effective in fighting diseases such as malaria, polio, and influenza. Their antibiotics were more efficient in fighting infections. But the same hospitals and Western medicines and procedures brought about the death of the African imagination in the field of medicine. Since the use of African medicines was discouraged by Christian preachers, the traditional medical practitioners ran short of patients. Consequently, most of them stopped researching and experimenting with traditional medicines and rituals. David Livingstone despised the Bakuena rain doctor for charming the clouds with medicines to persuade them to provide rain. However, almost the same method is used by Western scientists to do cloud seeding in order to charm the clouds to produce rain. So, it can be argued that African traditional scientists could perform cloud seeding before the Western scientists discovered it. The African medical research was stifled, and it died a premature death because of the criticism and the hate levelled against it. In recent years, some Christian churches in Zimbabwe have started encouraging their followers to use traditional herbs. They have established herbal gardens, which are run by Christians in which they grow oriental and Western herbs. This noble idea has come too late because most African Christians have lost the knowledge of their own healing herbs. Very few people cared to learn the art of healing because it was considered evil. My grandmother's sister, Mai Zhezha, was a renowned n'anga, but no one in our family tried to learn a thing from her until she died. Her medical wisdom and expertise of the life-giving herbs and rituals were lost when she died.

Although most of the rich Shona people who had accepted Christianity turned their backs to the traditional medicines, most of the poor

---

10. The conversation between the medical doctor and the rain doctor that has been quoted above.

people who lived in the rural areas continued to rely on *n'angas*. One of the reasons for the tenacity of this relationship was economic. Some people failed to raise bus fares to visit the mission hospitals, most of which treated the patients for free. Despite being Christians, they used what was closer to them—the *n'angas*. Some rich people too had one leg in the traditional medical field and the other in the Western, and it has remained like that up to this day. When things are alright, most people stick with the Western medicines. But, when people encounter medical complications or misfortunes that the Western medical practitioners cannot understand and cure, they turn to African medicines. Some people take medicines from both worlds at the same time. Although hospitals do not allow this dual medication, patients still do it without the knowledge of the nurses and doctors. Some *n'angas* also encourage the use of both medicines. I remember accompanying my mother to a *n'anga* because my nephew was sick. The *n'anga* performed the rituals that were intended to exorcize him of the evil spirits that were believed to have assaulted him. After performing all her rituals, the *n'anga* encouraged my mother to take my nephew to the hospital where he could have blood transfusion, if deemed necessary. Most *n'angas* refer their patients to hospitals, although nurses and doctors do not refer any of their patients to *n'angas*.

The condemnation of *n'angas* and traditional medicines has led to the need for African-style healing in mainline churches. Some pastors in mainline churches have responded positively by performing faith healing for their followers despite the condemnation from the official teachings of their churches. In Zambia, Archbishop Emmanuel Mlingo performed faith healing until he was whisked to the Vatican, where he ended up leaving the Roman Catholic Church. In Zimbabwe, the Roman Catholic Church produced Father Augustine Urayai, who performed faith healing and exorcisms. At some point in his ministry, he was suspended from active ministry, only to be reinstated by the late Bishop of Gweru, Tobias Wunganai Chiginya.[11] Although many Catholics respected Fr. Urayai's ministry, he never gained much support from his colleagues until his death.

The Anglican Church in Zimbabwe produced Father Lazarus Muyambi, who founded Chita Chezvipo Zvemoto (CZM) Primary School, Gokwe St Agnes Children's Home, Healing School and a girls' high boarding

---

11. In 1997, as part of the fulfillment of the Bachelor of Arts Honors in Religious Studies at the University of Zimbabwe, I visited Fr. Augustine Urayai at Chinyuni Mission, where he was the parish priest. I stayed with him for a week and listened to his views about evil spirits and healing. He strongly believed that witchcraft was a reality, and that ancestors were evil. He performed exorcism in most of his long Masses. I also witnessed some Catholics visiting Father Urayai for healing.

school. One thing that is common to the mainline churches' faith healing activities is that the causes of illness and misfortunes are similar to the African traditional causes. The difference lays in the medical interventions that they prescribe. The pastors use holy water, prayers, crosses, crucifixes, medals, novenas, and other religious sacred objects, whereas *n'angas* use water, herbs, animals, chickens, among others.

The Shona people who feel that the mainline churches are too patronizing concerning faith healing, use the services of the African Independent Churches prophets. These prophets diagnose the same causes of sickness as *n'angas*. Some members of the mainline churches visit them secretly whenever misfortunes that have an African flavor visit them. Some African Christians shuttle between hospitals, *n'angas*, prophets, and their own churches. It seems that the modern prophets have borrowed a lot from the traditional medical practitioners, including some of their healing methods. Their philosophy and theology will be explored in the next chapter.

The current relationship between Christianity and the traditional medical fraternity is not cordial. In Zimbabwe, the *n'angas* established an association, the Zimbabwe National Traditional Healers Association (ZINATHA) to harmonize their activities, share ideas and expertise, and to make members accountable for any wayward behavior, but this did not help in removing the stigma from this noble profession. Although the advent of Western medicines benefited Africans, it suffocated the research and experiments by *n'angas*, for they were starved of patients. Many Africans shied away from learning the traditional art of healing, and thus, the medical traditions that Africans had amassed from time immemorial were lost. It is too late now for Christian pastors and Westerners to turn around and say that herbs are good. What does it profit a people to lose the knowledge of home grown, life-giving herbs, yet grasping herbs without African names from the Orient or Europe?

9

African Independent Churches

Anyone who has a religious instinct cannot avoid noticing them under trees, on top of hills, alongside Zimbabwe's roads, in buses, at funerals and weddings, in their houses and open-air worshiping spaces, and almost everywhere. These are the ubiquitous, white-clad *Mapositori* (Apostles), multi-colored *Mazioni* (Zionists), and the professionally dressed Pentecostal Christians. The Roman Catholic Church's dream that one day all the straying and protesting children of God, who are members of the so-called *sects*, would be converted and be brought back to the true fold, has died a slow but sure death. These so-called *sects*, which contemporary scholars respectfully call African Independent Churches (AICs), have come to stay, and many members of the mainline Christian churches in Africa, either openly or in secret, heed their call.[1] Most of these African Independent Churches recruit their members from the mainline churches, to the chagrin of the leadership of the affected churches.

There are two scenarios concerning the attitude of the members of the mainline churches who attend African Independent Churches. On the one hand, some Christians have decided to leave their original churches, to become unwavering cardholding members of AICs. In fact, some of them have become serious critics of their original mainline churches. Some pastors use the testimonies of such born-again Christians as evidence of the uselessness of the abandoned churches. On the other hand, some Christians have one leg in some mainline church and another in some AIC. Some of these Christians attend their original church worship in the morning, and then rush for another church service in one of the AICs, in the afternoon. This dual religious allegiance has become a significant challenge to the mainline churches' leadership in Zimbabwe. Some scholars have interpreted this multiple religiosity as a sign of some theological and pastoral deficiency in the mainline churches.

The proclivity of many pastors who are faced with such a challenge is to blame and chastise those so-called lost souls, and demonize the AICs with

1. Mainline/mission churches are the major missionary churches that include The Roman Catholic Church, Reformed Church in Zimbabwe, Anglican Church, Methodist Church, Lutheran Church, and many others.

which their lost flocks flirt. Most of the time, the pastors' chastisement is not successful in changing the minds and hearts of the Christians who have a divided allegiance. The tendency to blame and castigate these double-faced Christians alone for this situation, without the concerned pastors performing a balanced examination of the factors that promote this behavior, shows how myopic some pastors are. Very few pastors who encounter such an exodus of their parishioners ever perform a self-examination, just in case they are the ones causing the exodus. Every caring pastor should investigate the causes of such an exodus, even if some of the causes might point at the pastor's own deficiencies as the leader of the flock.

Origins and Typology

Let us start from the beginning. In Zimbabwe, African Independent Churches came into existence in the twentieth century as a religious import from South Africa. These churches have been derogatorily called prophetic movements, messianic movements, millennial movements, nativistic movements, syncretistic movements, witchcraft eradication movements, revival movements, and separatist movements.[2] Some of these churches have fired back at their critics by pointing at their shortcomings. Hence, the Roman Catholic Church has been described as devilish, Satanist, and just a mere organization headed by the Anti-Christ. There is a huge mutual antagonism and condemnation between African Independent Churches and mainline churches. However, some progressive scholars of religion have positively named these churches, African Independent Churches, African Initiated Churches, or African Indigenous Churches. Whatever people may call them, many mainline church leaders have come to realize that AICs are a force to reckon with, have come to stay, and should never be taken for granted.

Harold Turner has defined African Independent Churches as churches that were "founded in Africa by Africans and primarily for Africans."[3] His definition is still significant today because most members of such churches are Africans, although some of the churches have members from other racial groups as well. Just to expand Harold Turner's definition, AICs are churches that were founded *in* Africa, *by* Africans, and primarily *for* Africans, for the purpose of transforming the lives of their adherents, through the interpretation and application of the Hebrew Scriptures and the message of Jesus Christ, in a manner that is consistent with the Afri-

---

2. Barrett, *Schism and Renewal in Africa*, 47–49.
3. Turner, *African Independent Church*, 92.

can worldview and context. This African context includes: values, culture, customs, morality, politics, economics, and beliefs, among other things. The founders of these churches realized that the universality of the message of Jesus Christ, did not imply a homogenous way of evangelization, but unity in diversity. They respect the fact that the Christian gospel comes to a people that already has a culture and religion that shape the way they understand and interpret their experiences. Every new experience, including the message of Christianity, has to be scrutinized using the same cultural and religious frameworks.

Typology

The oldest typology of AICs was done by Bengt B. M. Sundkler, in his 1941-book, *Bantu Prophets in South Africa*. He classified these churches into two major typologies, namely, *Ethiopian* and *Zionist*. Ethiopian churches are the ones that came out of the mission churches because of one reason or another, and were founded by Africans. Their earliest slogan was "Africa for Africans," which had political overtones. The earliest of Ethiopian churches came into being in the late nineteenth and early twentieth centuries when most Africans were beginning to resent the way Christianity was used as a vanguard for European imperialism and patronage. Most of Ethiopian churches kept the "fundamental doctrinal essence, organizational rules, and priestly forms" of their mother churches.[4] For Harold W. Turner, the dominant motive in the earliest secessions was the quest for spiritual independency, "rather than any quarrel with the orthodox practices or opinions of the older churches."[5] Some of the earliest Ethiopian-type churches in South Africa were: Zulu Mbiyana Church (1890), The Ethiopian Church (1892), Zulu Congregational Church (1896), Presbyterian Church of Africa (1898), African Mission Home Church (1907), African United Zulu Church (1916), African Congregational Church (1917), Zulu of African Ethiopian Church (1918), and others. The earliest Ethiopian-type AICs to come to Zimbabwe was the First Ethiopian Church, founded by Mupambi Chidembo, in 1910.[6]

Ethiopia was a very appealing name to the founders of AICs because of three primary reasons. First, Ethiopia is one of the few African countries that are mentioned in the Bible. There are over seventy passages in the Bible that refer to either Ethiopia or Cush. Second, Ethiopia and Liberia are the only African countries that were never or not quite colonized by the European

---

4. Sundkler, *Bantu Prophets in South Africa*, 54.
5. Turner, *History of an African Independent Church, Vols. 1–2*, 5.
6. Daneel, *Quest for Belonging*, 51.

powers. The Italian attempt to colonize Ethiopia in the late nineteenth century was not quite successful after King Menelik II's army defeated the Italians at the Battle of Odowa, in 1896. For many Africans, Ethiopia was a symbol of Black resistance, sovereignty, territorial integrity, and empowerment. Third, the Rastafari Movement that claims Marcus Garvey as its founder, started in Jamaica in the 1930s, also did popularize Ethiopia by claiming that it was the original home of all Africans and was the new Zion to which all Black people in the diaspora were supposed to be repatriated. They also taught that King Haile Selassie I of Ethiopia, who ascended the throne in 1930, was the incarnate of God. Some scholars are of the opinion that Ethiopia was probably a name used for Africa in the biblical era.

Bengt G. M. Sundkler named the second group of AICs, *Zionist*. Some of the earliest churches of this nomenclature had the word *Zionist, Apostolic, Pentecostal*, and others, in their names, and had their roots in Zion City of Illinois, USA.[7] They emphasized the works of the Holy Spirit, and strongly believed in miraculous healing, speaking in tongues, faith healing, and ritual purification.[8] According to Inus Daneel, these Spirit-type AICs are more recent than the Ethiopian-type.[9] In his 1961 edition of the same book, Sundkler added a third type, which he christened, *Messianic*, and referring to those churches whose leaders were respected by their followers as if they were Christ. It should be noted that very few church founders ever claimed to be Christ or equal to Christ, hence Inus Daneel encourages extreme caution when applying this term.[10] However, he observes that the reverence and mystical powers accorded to some AICs founders are elevated to the messianic level. For instance, "By the start of the 1990s (Ezekiel) Guti was subject to a great deal of reverence and adoration. He was addressed in praise names: Apostle, Servant of God, and the Man of God."[11] His followers are said to have prayed to the God of Guti.[12]

Sundkler might have had in mind other AICs leaders such as Prophet Simon Kimbangu, who founded The Church of the Lord Jesus Christ on Earth, in 1921, in Kinshasa, Zaire, whose followers revered him as if he were Christ. Harold W. Turner encourages scholars of AICs to cease the use of the term *Messianic* in reference to some founders of AICs because very few

---

7. Sundkler, *Bantu Prophets in South Africa*, 54
8. Daneel, *Quest for Belonging*, 39.
9. Ibid., 40.
10. Ibid., 42.
11. Maxwell, *African Gifts of the Spirit*, 138.
12. Ibid., 139.

leaders do qualify for that typology.[13] Although the Sundkler typology helps researchers in categorizing these churches, most researchers agree that it is a very difficult task to find an inclusive typology for all of AICs because of their tremendous number and diversity. According to Martin West, in 1970, there were over 3,000 AICs in South Africa alone.[14] The rate at which they are founded has increased in the past decades.

African Independent Churches in Zimbabwe

Let us come closer home. The earliest African Independent Churches came to Zimbabwe through South Africa. These were: Zion Christian Church of Bishop Samuel Mutendi of Bikita, the Zion Apostolic Church of South Africa, led by Bishop David Masuka, and Zion Apostolic Faith Mission of Bishop Andreas Shoko.[15] The last two are called Zioni *retambo/ndaza*, which refers to the sacred thread that the followers of these churches tie around their wrists or waists to protect themselves from evil spirits. Both Andreas Shoko and Samuel Mutendi had joined Lekhanyane Enginasi's Zion Apostolic Faith Mission in South Africa, where they worked as bricklayers, and when Enginasi formed the Zion Christian Church, Samuel Mutendi joined.[16] Daneel says that David Masuka, Mtisi, and Makamba, joined bishop Mhlangu's Zion Apostolic Church of South Africa and were baptized in the "Jordan."[17] Other churches followed. Johane Masowe, born Shoniwa Masedza Tandi Moyo, started the Gospel of God Church in the 1930s. Mutumwa (Apostle) Paul Mwazha, whose message sounded both Ethiopian and Zionist, founded the African Apostolic Church in 1951.

As of today, hundreds of African Independent Churches have mushroomed in Zimbabwe. In 1995, it was believed that 50 percent of Christians in Zimbabwe belonged to African Independent Churches.[18] Some of the latest and most popular African Independent Churches in Zimbabwe are: Worldwide Family of God of Prophet of Andrew Wutawunashe (1980), Zimbabwe Assemblies of God (ZAOGA) of Apostle Ezekiel Guti (1960), The Prophetic Healing Deliverance (PHD) of the controversial Prophet Walter Magaya (2012), and The United Family International Church (UFIC) of Prophet Emmanuel Makandiwa and Prophetess Ruth Makandiwa. UFIC

13. Turner, *Religious Innovation in Africa*, 53.
14. West, *Bishops and Prophets in a Black City*, 1.
15. Bucher, *Spirits and Power*, 130.
16. Ibid., 132.
17. Daneel, *Old and New in Southern Shona Independent Churches Vol. 1*, 289.
18. Cox, *Fire from Heaven*, 245.

is one of the latest churches in Zimbabwe that have taken Christianity by storm. It was founded in August 2008, at the Anglican Cathedral in Harare, and was officially launched in 2010. Its mission statement summarizes what it stands for: "To unite the body of Jesus Christ (the Church) through reaching out to the lost, the poor, the less privileged members of the society, widows, orphans and the broken hearted, ultimately imparting revelation knowledge of Jesus Christ and fellowshipping with God the Father, God the Son and God the Holy Spirit."[19] The main venue of this Church in Harare is the City Sports Center, but they are constructing a 30,000-seater auditorium in Chitungwiza. UFIC is one of the fastest growing churches in Zimbabwe. In the 2014 edition of the Judgement Night, about 70 000 UFIC congregants gathered at the National Sports Stadium in Harare.[20] Thousands of the followers of this Church converge at the City Sports Center in Harare every Tuesday and Sunday for services. Some of the adherents belong to other Christian denominations, and still confess to be members of their original churches. It has since spread to all cities in Zimbabwe, and has even crossed the border into South Africa. UFIC, like other Christian churches of its nature, emphasizes the message of prosperity, healing, exorcism, and the performance of miracles.

Worldview and Liturgy

Most of the AICs in Zimbabwe share a common worldview. Their liturgy has praise and worship, which involves the singing of hymns, praying, and dancing. Some AICs have choirs and bands that lead the singing. Usually the songs are choruses that can easily be learnt by the adherents and visitors. Some AICs punctuate the singing with spirited dances and prayers in which the followers may cry or laugh in the spirit. Some may speak in tongues. The praise and worship is followed by the liturgy of the word in which the pastor gives a long homily either in vernacular or English. If the homily is in English, there is usually a translator. Healing and deliverance may follow the homily. Sick members of the congregation are invited to come forward where they stand in a line waiting for their turn to be prayed for by the pastors. It is during this time when demons are exorcized. Immediately after the healing, testimonies of God's work among the congregants may be shared. After the testimonies, pledges of tithes may be made and offerings collected.

19 UFIC official webpage, http://www.ufiministries.org/index.php/features/about-ufi, accessed on 10/27/2016.

20. Pindula, http://www.pindula.co.zw/United_Family_International_Church, accessed on 10/27/2016.

One of the central practice of these churches is the all-night prayer or night vigils, which Titus Leonard Presler, who traces their history and development to African Traditional Religion, and the Liberation Struggle of Zimbabwe, believes them to be ". . . central in spirit possession, in the initiation of spirit mediums, in funerals and in subsequent propitiatory rites, often with the ceremonial climax occurring just before dawn."[21] Some churches hold such night vigils once every week, and others hold them less frequently. The night vigils have also been borrowed by guild members of the mainline churches though at a less frequent rate. The vigils are primarily for prayers, singing, testimonies, and dancing. Presler thinks that the night is favored by both Christians and traditionalists in Zimbabwe because it is a conducive time of spiritual power in which spirits can easily be accessed since they do wander around during this time.[22] The Shona call these night vigils, *pungwe*, which means to spend the whole night awake.

Reasons for Proliferation

One of the questions that many researchers have asked is why such churches can attract thousands of followers within such a short period. One of the most interesting attempts to give a rationale behind the successes of these churches comes from F. B. Welbourn and B. A. Ogot's book, *A Place to Feel at Home* that was published in 1966. According to the two scholars, Africans wanted a mental dwelling place in which they would feel at home. That dwelling placing had been denied them in the mainline churches for many years. Almost everything in the mission churches was too strange for Africans to derive comfort from it. Most of the priests in mainline churches were Whites, who struggled to preach in vernacular. Some of them did master the languages of the people that they served, but preaching in such languages was not easy. Those who preached in English needed translators, and that made the service too long for the people's comfort. More so, during the early days of Christianity in Zimbabwe, translators were hard to find.

The mission churches' liturgy was very strange to most Africans, too. The Roman Catholic Church Mass was celebrated in Latin, a language that most Catholics did not understand. The tunes of the songs that they sang were too artificial, and sometimes very difficult to learn. The African drums and jingles were initially forbidden by some mainline churches. Up to now, one needs a hymnbook to be able to join others in singing in some of the

---

21. Presler, *Transfigured Night*, 13.
22. Ibid., 57, 64.

mainline churches. Singing from a book was unfamiliar to Africans because Africans did not have hymn books during their traditional liturgies.

In the Roman Catholic Church, new song compositions keep coming year after year to the extent that it becomes so hard to keep pace with the new tunes. One can easily become a stranger in her own father's house, in the Roman Catholic Church, in Zimbabwe. Dancing in church during official rituals was either banned or controlled. The African kind of dance was castigated for being too vigorous, and sometimes sensual, and therefore, undignified for sacred gatherings. The Roman Catholic Church later allowed a slight movement of the body and feet as acceptable and dignified dancing during Mass. Consequently, most African Christians had two types of dances, one for the church and the other for secular celebrations in their homes.

To worsen the matter, the biblical passages that the pastors read for the parishioners each Sunday were prescribed by the top leaders of the church, most of the time, without any consideration of the people's context. The Christian worldview was foreign, and that resulted in the message of the pastors' homilies being irrelevant to most of the listeners. For many Africans, what happened in the church was very different from how Africans lived in their homes. The church was so divorced from the African ways of doing things. In the end, some Africans refused to join mainline churches, and chose to stay in their traditional ways. Some of those who converted, remained sitting on the fence, with one leg in the mainline church, and the other, in the African Traditional Religion.

The leaders of AICs accurately read the situation, and founded churches that provided Africans what was lacking in the mission churches. They ordained Africans as pastors, and availed preaching and liturgical services in vernacular. Those changes enhanced the people's understanding of the gospel message. They allowed the singing of choruses that were easier to learn, and by so doing encouraged the active participation of all the people of God. They selected relevant and contextual readings from the Bible, which the audience could apply to their lives. They allowed the African dancing styles during liturgy. The AICs indeed minimized the dichotomy between the secular and the Christian lives. This relevance and contextuality continue to draw people to AICs at the expense of mainline churches today. In Zimbabwe, founders such as Johane Maranke, Ezekiel Guti, Mai Chaza, Andrew Wutaunashe, Walter Magaya, Emmanuel Makandiwa, and many others, observed what the people lacked, and provided it in their churches.

Sundkler thinks that the proliferation of AICs was exacerbated by the nineteenth century socio-economic factors in South Africa. The economic boom that South Africa experienced starting from 1885 when diamonds were discovered at Kimberly, and later, when gold was discovered in the

Witwatersrand, brought people from all over Africa to work in the mines in South Africa.[23] The journey to South Africa was long, perilous, and lonely. Consequently, most migrant workers went to South Africa without their families. Away from the comfort of their homes, cultures, families, and relatives, most migrant workers felt lonely, and at times, alienated. The mission churches, some of which segregated against Africans, had no consolation to extend to these migrant workers. A remedy was provided by AICs, which gave them a second family, and indeed a place to feel at home, far away from home. Racial segregation, which unfortunately found its way into the mission churches, and was sometimes propagated by their pastors, drove some Africans away from such churches. The apartheid that had been established by the Whites as soon as they settled in South Africa, and was upgraded through the Native Land Act of 1913, and Urban Areas Act of 1923, and the heavy taxation of Africans, further alienated and impoverished Blacks.[24] The founders of African Independent Churches in South Africa took advantage of the situation, and provided Blacks with a warm home where they could contextualize the message of Jesus to console and offer them hope, song, and drums to dance away their loneliness.

The other important factor that led to the proliferation of AICs was the condemnation of the African culture by the missionaries. For most missionaries, African culture was barbaric, primitive, superstitious, and archaic. They condemned the veneration of the ancestors, a condemnation which was tantamount to an "onslaught on the very foundations of the African Tribal and family structure."[25] In Zimbabwe, the missionaries desecrated the Matopos Hills, which were the headquarters of the Shona God, Mwari. Furthermore, some of the missionaries seemed to be on the side of witches, by denouncing the traditional medical practitioners. African names, songs, dances, drums, and other musical instruments were condemned. They also condemned polygamy, and refused to baptize husbands, wives, and children who belonged to polygamous families. Those Christians "who lapsed into polygamy were excommunicated or otherwise disciplined."[26] Many Africans who could not stomach the above humiliation moved to AICs. For example, the African National Church in Malawi was founded in 1929 to take care of polygamists. Its founder, Simon Kamkhati Mkandawire was a polygamist who had been expelled from the Livingstonia Church in 1914. In 1928, with the support of his polygamist friends and former graduates of Livingstonia

23. Sundkler, *Bantu Prophets in South Africa*, 27.
24. Ibid., 33–34.
25. Daneel, *Quest for Belonging*, 74.
26. Barrett, *Schism and Renewal in Africa*, 117.

Mission, he founded The African National Church.[27] His church catered for the Africans who had the same grievances as his.

Some early missionaries were accused of failing to eradicate witchcraft, and to perform faith healing. Africans lived in perpetual fear of evil spirits and witches. They expected missionaries to deal with that problem since they had condemned the traditional medical practitioners, who had up to that point, protected them from the baneful activities of evil spirits and witches. Unfortunately, the missionaries, either discouraged witchcraft beliefs by ignoring them, or supported the colonial governments' endeavor to quash them through legislation. As if that was not bad enough, the hospitals that the missionaries established did not take care of the illnesses that were believed to have been caused by witchcraft. In addition, mission hospitals did not provide their patients with the causes of sickness that were compatible with the African worldview. Furthermore, Africans were introduced to natural causes of diseases, which many accepted, but did not fully understand. Most Africans were convinced that insects such as mosquitoes could cause the deadly Malaria, but no sufficient explanation was given as to why the treacherous mosquito would choose to bite a particular person, and not the other, at any given time. Likewise, their experiences had taught them that some women would die of childbirth complications, and they knew the reasons for that. The hospital staff gave them explanations that were incompatible with their philosophy. Most Africans believed that they knew the causes of most misfortunes—witchcraft, but the missionaries discouraged them from believing that.

The founders of AICs were different. They explained the causes of diseases in a manner that was intelligible to the African mind. Most of these churches did exorcize people of witchcraft and healed the sick from its effects. Often, some of the people who confessed to missionaries that they were witches wanted to get rid of their bewitching concoctions, but most missionaries did not want to be involved. Some of those people joined AICs. Even those people who remained in mission churches, at times visited the AICs whenever necessity demanded it. In Zimbabwe, most of the Apostolic Churches make it their central mission to eradicate witchcraft, and heal their followers of its effects. Of course, most of the AICs condemn traditional medical practitioners and their healing methods, but they have maintained the same worldview concerning the causes of diseases. Some of them forbid their followers from using European medicines as well.

It is argued that the need for leadership opportunities forced some Africans to found their own churches. At that time, most African nations

27. Ranger, *The African Churches of Tanzania*, 16–20.

had been conquered, and were being ruled by European powers. Most of their leaders had been stripped of their authority and power by the colonizers. There were many talented Africans who could have become secular leaders, but the opportunities were so slim. Some of the people who converted to the mission churches saw it as an opportunity to showcase their leadership qualities. Some of them had worked tirelessly side by side with the missionaries as catechists, and even surpassed many missionaries in the business of winning souls for God. However, most of these assistants' leadership abilities were never acknowledged by their masters. The only way for them to receive recognition as leaders was to start their own churches in which discipline was not imposed from abroad. This way, they managed to practice the leadership skills that they had acquired from working with the missionaries.[28]

Some scholars have argued that one of the major causes of the proliferation of AICs was the success of the missionaries. The missionaries preached the word of God, and Africans understood their message to the extent of starting their own churches. By starting their own churches, they were displaying the profundity of their understanding of the word of God that had been passed on to them by the missionaries. This scenario is normal in life. Let us take the example of a classroom practitioner. Most teachers are happy when their students understand what they are taught, and more are happier when their students become better than the teachers themselves. Similarly, a mother rejoices when her daughter becomes a better mother than herself. Some scholars think that the same mentality should be applied to religion. The multiplication of AICs should be a cause for jubilation by the mainline churches from which they would have graduated. Competitions for souls, and the blasphemous idea that only one religion possesses the totality of the salvific graces of God, prevent most church leaders to rejoice when more churches are established. Be that as it may, several pastors of the mission churches argue that the founding of new churches by Africans is a sign of the lack of understanding of the message of Christ. For them, it is only their form of Christianity that is acceptable to God, and anyone who starts his own church would have failed to understand their message.

In the beginning of mainline Christianity in Africa, only the missionary could read and interpret the Bible for their congregants because most Africans were illiterate. Even when they started to receive Western education, most Africans still had difficulties in understanding the English language in which the Bible was written. The missionaries could read the Greek and Hebrew Bibles, and that gave them absolute control over the

---

28. Ranger, *The African Churches of Tanzania*, 10.

scriptures.[29] Eventually, the Bible was translated into vernacular, and many people could now read it for themselves. In their virgin exploration of the Bible, some Africans are reported to have discovered that the missionary had read the Bible selectively. They stumbled on very important passages, which the missionary had not read for them. For instance, they discovered that polygamy, an African practice that missionaries had relentlessly and unsparingly attacked, was also practiced in the biblical times. Abraham, Moses, Jacob, King David, and many other biblical figures that are said to have lived exemplary lives were indeed polygamous.[30] King Solomon, who is considered to be one of the wisest kings ever to grace the Jewish nation, had seven hundred official wives and three hundred concubines. For some Africans, it seemed as though the missionaries only read the biblical passages that supported their own cultural values, and ignored those passages that supported the African culture, despite the fact that the same missionaries claimed that the entire Bible was the inspired word of God. To some Africans, the selective reading of biblical passages by missionaries was tantamount to conspiracy and hypocrisy.

Some of the above reasons are still the pushing factors for people who leave the mainline churches for AICs. Most leaders of AICs accurately diagnose the needs of the members of mainline churches and other Africans, and promise to resolve them in their new churches. First, they preach the gospel of prosperity and hope to an audience that has lost hope of ever achieving these in the mission churches. Africans, by their very nature and tradition, pray for prosperity, which they intend to achieve here on earth. Although most mission churches promised their followers the achievement of that prosperity through the establishment of their mission schools, these increasingly became more expensive, and far beyond the reach of many ordinary Africans. The economic prospects of most African countries paint a gloomy picture for ordinary citizens' economic aspirations. In Zimbabwe, the unemployment rate is over 80 percent, and some people have turned to AICs for consolation. AICs do not give people jobs, but their pastors show that they care for their followers by talking and praying about jobs and prosperity. Their message keeps people going, living one day at a time.

The need for faith healing and its promise by the leaders of the AICS is another "effective evangelistic instrument for preaching the good news to the African poor."[31] One of the soteriological beliefs of traditional Africans is the relentless pursuit of good health. Due to the economic stress that the

29. Barrett, *Schism and Renewal in Africa*, 127.
30. Daneel, *Quest for Belonging*, 84.
31. Anderson, *Zion and Pentecost*, 125.

country is experiencing, many Zimbabweans cannot afford the service of Western physicians. Consequently, some people have turned to faith healing. In his book, *Zionism and Faith-Healing in Rhodesia,* 1970, M. L. Daneel has explored the type of healing that Africans seek from AICs, particularly the Zion Christian Church of Samuel Mutendi. Some of the issues for which members of AICs seek healing are like those the traditional Shona sought for help from the traditional medical practitioners. For instance, adherents of AICs use the services of their pastors and prophets for healing from barrenness or the predetermination of the sex of unborn children.[32] Although some pastors in the mainline churches pray for the sick members of their congregations, they never make it an integral and regular part of their liturgy. Some of those who do pray for the sick members of their congregations, do not take the healing apostolate seriously. In fact, some of them do not even believe in the efficacy of healing prayers.

Leaders of the AICs consider healing as one of the most critical aspects of their worship. Martin West has categorized their healing into three parts, namely, healing during church services, healing by immersion, and healing that is performed by a prophet after being consulted by the sick person.[33] Healing during church services is performed every time the congregation gathers for worship as has been described above. Healing by immersion is performed at the *Jordan River* in which the sick members are completely immersed in sacred water.[34] The immersion is believed to cast out evil spirits that cause sickness. The healing by consultation of the prophet is done by individual members who feel the need to consult such prophets. The consultation may be done publicly in a church gathering or privately, at the healing center of the prophet. When AICs prophets pray for the sick, the energy and time that they invest to it show the level of faith they have in the therapeutic power of prayer. In addition to prayers for healing, they also pray for the frustration of the machinations of the evil spirits and witches. They claim to cast them to arid places where they perish of thirst and heat.

Longevity has always been one of the ultimate pursuit of the traditional Africans. This longevity can be achieved either by an individual or a family. AICs are deeply concerned with the same longevity. The people whose lives have been cut short by the failure to beget children are likely to join the AICs so that their barrenness may be remedied. Lately, there has been talk of miracle babies in Zimbabwe that are conceived through the intervention

---

32. Daneel, *Zionism and Faith-Healing in Rhodesia*, 30.

33. West, *Bishops and Prophets in a Black City*, 92.

34. The *Jordan River* refers to any river that a particular AIC leader chooses to perform rituals such as baptism and other ritual cleansings.

of pastors and prophets' prayers. The need to have children in the African community is crucial, and many people are willing to do even the unthinkable for the sake of begetting children. There is no doubt that most pastors of the mainline churches possess the power to heal, but since most of them do not dedicate most of their time and energy to doing it, some of their followers seek healing from AICs that consider faith healing seriously.

Pope Francis has pointed out one of the most important challenges that may drive some Catholics out of the Roman Catholic Church, namely, the inadequate preparation for and delivery of homilies by some priests. He writes:

> Let us now look at preaching within the liturgy, which calls for serious consideration by pastors. I will dwell in particular, and even somewhat meticulously, on the homily and its preparation, since so many concerns have been expressed about this important ministry, and we cannot simply ignore them. The homily is the touchstone for judging a pastor's closeness and ability to communicate to his people. We know that the faithful attach great importance to it, and that both they and their ordained ministers suffer because of homilies: the laity from having to listen to them and the clergy from having to preach them! It is sad that this is the case. The homily can actually be an intense and happy experience of the Spirit, a consoling encounter with God's word, a constant source of renewal and growth.[35]

The Holy Father is right in saying that there are concerns about the quality of the homilies preached by some Roman Catholic priests, and that listening to some of them is painful. It seems that some priests do not adequately prepare for their homilies. The homilies of such priests lack depth, contextuality, and application. They leave the listeners in doubt concerning the relevant and practical application of their message. Sometimes the homilies sound beautiful, but lack guidelines in which the listeners may apply them to their daily struggles as members of the pilgrim church on this earth. To worsen the matter, most Roman Catholic priests do not solicit for feedback from the parishioners concerning their homilies. The Holy Father thinks that some ministers do not adequately prepare for homilies. Preparation involves the consultation of biblical commentaries, knowledge of the context of the parishioners, an inspiring reading of the word of God, and a passionate and prophetic delivery of the homily.

---

35. Pope Francis, *Apostolic Exhortation Evangelii Gaudium*, Chapter 3, Section II, para. 135, November 24, 2013.

There are other several issues that may contribute to the delivery of poor homilies by some pastors. First, the criteria for becoming a Roman Catholic priest focus on academic brilliance and one's aptitude for celibate life, among other things. However, there is no question asked about the talent and willingness of the seminarian to learn how to prepare and deliver inspiring homilies. Of course, many seminaries offer homiletics as one of the courses that seminarians should study, but whatever happens to the mastered skills after seminary is hard to know. Second, although the Roman Catholic liturgy is divided into two major parts, there has been a tendency to overemphasize the liturgy of the Eucharist at the expense of the liturgy of the Word. The priest knows that most Catholics are contented with receiving Holy Communion more than hearing the word of God. He knows that many Catholics can tolerate half-baked holies, as long as they are not starved of the Holy Communion.

Third, the Roman Catholic clergy are not hired by the parishioners, but are assigned to parishes by the bishops. Hence, most of them, if not all, do not worry about looking for a job. They are not affected by the stiff competition that may come from other job seekers because almost every diocese has a shortage of priests. If Roman Catholic priests were interviewed, hired, and fired by the parishioners for negligence of duty or the failure to perform, most priests would take homilies seriously. Moreover, Roman Catholic priests inherit parishes that were established by other priests, missionaries, or catechists, and some of them never feel the need to attract more people to their parishes than they find in those parishes. For some pastors, the winning of souls for God is the work of catechists and other religious education teachers. They come, stay, and leave the parish the way it was when they arrived. In fact, some priests would make sure that by the time they leave the parish, their poor and atrocious homilies would have driven some parishioners away.

Most AICs pastors do not have that luxury since most of them must start from scratch if they are founders of a church. Some of them must compete for the few posts that are available in their churches, and when they get the job, they should deserve their salaries by giving homilies that spiritually benefit their pay-givers. Some of these pastors are not as educated as the Roman Catholic priests, but they do better in terms of homilies. Sometimes one cannot avoid to bemoan the money and time used in training a Roman Catholic priest, after listening to his pathetic homilies. However, it should be noted that there are thousands of talented, inspiring, and diligent Roman Catholic preachers, the world over. The challenge that Catholics face is that such priests may not be in every parish.

Fourth, some Roman Catholic priests are cushioned from the life of the ordinary Christians right from the moment they get into seminary. Although they are of this world, they do not quite belong to the world, for the seminary life separates them from ordinary people. Some of them have lost touch with reality—the daily struggles that ordinary Christians encounter, and the burdens that they shoulder throughout the week. Some priests do not realize that when the people come for Mass on Sunday, it does not mean that they have nothing else to do, but they come so that the man of the cloth would use the word of God, to take off from their shoulders some of those burdens, to enable them to begin the new week feeling refreshed. In Zimbabwe, most of the newly ordained priests get a car, a house, and a job on the day of the ordination or soon thereafter. Some have never experienced the heart-rending and nerve-racking hunt for a job. They do not have a family to which they are directly responsible although some may support their parents and siblings. They do not have to struggle like the rest of the people to feed or take care of their sick children. It seems that some of them are deprived of the experiences of life that can teach someone to be humble, respectful, and preach from the heart.

Finally, as already mentioned, many Roman Catholic priests do not solicit for feedback on their homilies. To worsen the matter, parishioners are not free enough to offer that feedback voluntarily, particularly, if it is negative. The reason for the unwillingness to ask for feedback by the pastor may be a result of the fact that, in most countries, the Roman Catholic priest might be the only person in the parish who is theologically and philosophically literate. The difference between the levels of theological education between the Roman Catholic priest and most of his parishioners is alarming. It is a situation where a man with two university degrees, one in philosophy and the other in theology, preaches to barely catechized parishioners. Consequently, those Catholics who feel that their pastors' homilies do not deal with the challenges that they face daily in their communities, may end up leaving the Catholic Church, joining AICs. A good homily should show that the presenter knows the historical background of the biblical passage under interrogation, is aware of the past and contemporary scholarly interpretations of the same passage, can apply its message to his audience's *Sitz-im-Leben* (situation in life), and finally can challenge the audience to be transformed. A priest who knows his flock should be able to address each one of their needs using only one homily.

Another factor that pushes people from the Roman Catholic Church to AICs is the hypocrisy that is sometimes found in the pastors of the church in relation to the vow of chastity and celibacy. The priest is considered the model for a Christian life, and when he fails to fulfill that expectation, it scandalizes the people. Some of the sexual scandals that are perpetrated by some Roman Catholic priests betray the trust that parishioners have for them and their office. This expectation does not mean that ordinary people expect Roman Catholic priests to live like angels. Again, it does not mean that ordinary Christians are not involved in sexual scandals themselves. The difference between lay and ordained perpetrators of sexual misconduct is that the priest would have declared publicly that he has decided to forgo his sexual needs to serve the people of God. It is because of their willingness to embrace celibacy and chastity that they become default sacred practitioners of the Roman Catholic Church's rituals. That is why they are awarded the privileges to preside over the celebration of the Eucharist, baptism, and confessions of the people of God. Priests are not ordinary people. When they fail to keep their vows, it shakes the faith of many of their followers, and that may force some people to leave the Catholic Church.

Some people are drawn to AICs by the promise of the miraculous. Many founders of AICs claim to have the power to heal miraculously. They claim to have the powers to pray over barren women so that they may conceive. They claim to have the ability to make the disabled walk and the blind see. Some of them make it their business to pray for the unemployed members of their churches so that they can get jobs. They say they can cast out evil spirits that are believed to cause misfortunes, diseases, bad luck, and death. They talk of miracle babies and money. They claim to be able to make people lose weight. Although, it is difficult to prove that they can fulfill all those claims, the ordinary people believe them. It is true that there are many followers of these pastors whose prayers and wishes have not been met and will probably not be fulfilled in the future, but that does not deter them from following these churches. These pastors show that they are concerned about the needs of their followers, and by praying for them, they sustain their hopes of a better future. Hope gives many people a reason to live. It heals and transforms them.

Lessons for Mainline Churches

That AICs have come to stay is a fact that cannot be contested. Pope Francis acknowledges the challenges posed by "the proliferation of new religious movements, some of which tend to fundamentalism while others seem to propose a spirituality without God." The Holy Father thinks that "a predominantly individualistic culture," "unwelcoming atmosphere of some of our parishes and communities," and "the bureaucratic way of dealing with problems" are some of the contributing factors to that proliferation.[36] It should be noted that independent or non-denominational churches are all over the world, and that some of their pastors fish from mainline churches and from each other. The mainline churches need to do something about it. The Pope thinks that the evangelization of cultures by the gospel becomes an imperative that may remedy the situation. This evangelization involves: "encouraging, fostering and reinforcing a richness which already exists," "sparking new processes for evangelizing culture, and challenging "deficiencies which need to be healed by the Gospel: machismo, alcoholism, domestic violence, low Mass attendance, fatalistic or superstitious notions which lead to sorcery, and the like," while keeping in mind that "each culture and social group needs purification and growth."[37]

The lesson to be learned here is that Africans remain Africans even in the Christian churches. Africans can only receive the gospel as Africans and nothing else. Anyone who is serious about the genuine Christian conversion and the transformation of Africans should make the gospel applicable to their cultural context. Some theologians have suggested the implementation of inculturation that should start with the people. Inculturation should be spontaneous and a result of the promptings of the Holy Spirit, rather than an imposition from the top echelons of power. AICs have responded to the contextual and cultural needs of Zimbabweans. Their message is three-fold: the pursuit of prosperity here on earth, good health, and longevity. Whether their adherents get these or not is another thing. The fact that Prophet Emmanuel Makandiwa preaches about them is good enough for some followers. The Roman Catholic Church has to choose either to respond to the people's pursuit of the above needs, or fail to transform the people's faith and lives.

For most Africans, sickness threatens the attainment of prosperity, good health, and longevity, and therefore, it is the people's number one enemy. In the past, whenever somebody was ill, a holistic remedy was provided as soon as possible. Yes, mission churches built hospitals where many diseases are cured, but they have failed to explain the causes of these diseases in a manner that is intelligible to the African mind. They have also failed to heal certain diseases. They do not address the issue of evil forces and witchcraft. AICs take care of the above and some Africans have been consoled. Whether the healings that are witnessed on television are genuine or fake, it is neither here nor there. What is observed is a sincere need by Africans for faith

---

36. Pope Francis, *Apostolic Exhortation Evangelii Gaudium*, Chapter 2, Section I, para. 63, November 24, 2013.

37. Pope Francis, *Apostolic Exhortation Evangelii Gaudium*, Chapter 2, Section I, para., 69, November 24, 2013.

healing. When Christians read the Gospel, they find out that Jesus healed the sick and performed exorcisms. They expect their ministers to do the same. When this is not done, they go looking for them elsewhere. Now that the economic hardships Zimbabwe is facing make it extremely difficult for more and more people to pay their healthcare bills, people increasingly resort to the *prophets,* most of who are affordable, or do not charge any fee at all. The bottom line is that many Africans will understand no other gospel except the one that involves healing and exorcisms. If Catholic ministers continue to ignore or down-play that need, the faithful will continue to go elsewhere in search of health and wholeness. AICs are waiting for them.

One big sign concerning the need for miraculous healing by Catholics in Zimbabwe is seen in popular religiosity exhibited at the John Bradburne, Mutemwa Shrine. The people who have been there can bear witness to the fact that Roman Catholics are still Africans—very much in pursuit of prosperity, good health, and long life. What one sees there is a genuine thirst for healing that is Catholic in nature. Unfortunately, our pastors have not officially spoken concerning the devotions that are directed to that shrine.

Missionaries should be applauded for inculturating some aspects of the African culture. They allowed the singing of vernacular hymns, drumming, and dancing during liturgical celebrations. This development has been received well by most African Christians. However, there are a few challenges that need to be addressed. Some mainline churches' hymns are fixed, and most have been extracted from the Psalms. These hymns were composed for the Israelites, and were relevant to the Israelite context. Some of these hymns have become irrelevant to African believers because they were not composed for them. It is very surprising that church leaders think that hymns that were composed thousands of years ago, at a particular place, and for a specific people, may still be applicable to a different people, with a completely different context. Does it mean that African believers cannot reflect on the works of God among them, and be inspired to compose their own hymns? This observation does not mean that all biblical psalms are irrelevant to the Shona people's experiences, because some of them are still relevant.

More so, the hymns that are sung in the Roman Catholic Church in Zimbabwe have complicated tunes. It takes some practice to be able to sing them fluently and inspirationally. One hymn has many tunes. There are some Catholics who always remain strangers in their father's house. They cannot join others in singing because the tunes keep changing at a rate they cannot master. Now to deprive an African Christian of singing is tantamount to chasing her away from the church. Although AICs take some of their hymns from the Bible, they contextualize them. AICs sing choruses that can be learnt easily even by strangers. The tunes are vivid and contextual. Even Catholics buy these people's music DVDs, but members of AICs do not buy Catholic music. Whenever Catholics sing fast tune hymns, they are strongly reprimanded by their pastors and catechists. Those who want to feel at home as far as music is concerned should join AICs. One wonders if there is a musical tune that upsets God, and make the singers sinful.

Africans love to express themselves through dancing and most of them are great dancers. Fortunately, the RCC allows dancing, but a type of dancing that can be described as a mere movement. Shona Catholics have a dance for the church, and a different dance when they are at home. They are a divided people. Dancing during their worship is not inspiring for it is just a mere rhythmic movement. If Christianity is to become African and Africans Christian, true African dances should be allowed to take place in the church. If mainline churches fail to encourage them, some people will leave them and join the AICs where dancing is encouraged. In fact, AICs have given Christianity a unique African flavor.[38]

The Way Forward: Ongoing Formation and Ecumenism

If Catholics are to stay in the Catholic Church, some issues should be revisited. First, there should be an ongoing formation for all the Catholics. A prolific ongoing formation requires more teachers of faith who are qualified to do the job. The perennial shortage of priests ever since the coming of Catholicism to Africa has seen catechists working side by side with priests in teaching the faith. However, most of these well-intentioned teachers have not received proper training, and most of them work on voluntary basis. It seems that African catechists in Africa have been neglected by the Roman Catholic Church for a long time. Catechism is precious, and entrusting its instruction to an untrained and unpaid catechist is a gross violation of the rights of the people of God. If Catholics are to fully understand their faith, catechists should be theologically educated. One wonders why the parishioners do not demand at least five Ordinary Level passes or a Diploma in Theology/Religious Studies from anyone intending to teach catechism.

Catechetical institutions such as Wadzanai Training Center in Zimbabwe, have been training catechists for over two decades but most of its graduates have joined the Ministry of Education as teachers, in search of survival. Most of them are deterred from becoming full-time catechists because they will be asked to volunteer. Asking catechists to volunteer is

38. Anderson, *Zion and Pentecost*, 220.

one of the worst injustices the church has perpetrated and perpetuated in Africa. Most catechists do have families that need food on the table, and volunteering their skills may bring misery to their families. If the Catholic Church is serious about the quality of the people's faith, it should educate the catechists and pay them a reasonable remuneration. Catechesis should be transformed into a competitive profession, so that it begins to attract the best educated religious teachers. Volunteers are crucial in any field, but they should augment the efforts of trained and salaried catechists.

Second, the mainline churches should reform if they are to continue to be relevant to the needs of Africans, and to attract their undivided religious allegiance. They should learn how the AICs have managed to be so successful despite all the odds against them. They may learn a thing or two from the AICs, most of which have been fishing for converts from the mainline churches. Embarking on an honest dialogue with AICs may make that learning achievable and fruitful. This dialogue fosters mutual understanding and respect between the two groups. It is not helpful to perpetuate the historic mutual hatred and suspicion both groups, particularly Catholics and members of AICs, have for each other, because both are working in the vineyard of God to promote the transformation of God's people. It is the duty of all Christians to earnestly pursue the re-creation of a people acceptable to God and humanity.

Impediments and Common Grounds

However, dialogue is hampered by the mutual hatred and condemnation between Catholics and some members of AICs. The AICs condemn Catholics for drinking beer, eating pork and other forbidden foods, per the law of Moses. They derogatorily call Catholics, *vana Rambachawarutsa*, which means people who eat and drink everything. They castigate them for worshipping idols, referring to the many statues that are found in Catholic churches. Catholics are said to have no Holy Spirit, and hence, their inability to perform faith healing. They do not baptize their followers properly, in the Jordan River. Their singing is too artificial and out of context. They are also accused of worshiping the dead because of the Roman Catholic Church's inculturated burial rituals.

Catholics and members of the mainline churches condemn AICs for being syncretistic, which means the mixing of Christian and African Traditional Religious practices. Some Catholics and mainline churches members refuse to recognize these churches as Christian, but refer to them as sectarians. Their followers and leaders are derided for their illiteracy. They are also ridiculed for lacking sacraments and properly ordained clergy. The AICs' healing activities are sometimes condemned as stage-managed, fake, and misleading. Some of the AICs members are accused of abusing their children by preventing them from taking Western medicines. They are said to oppress, subjugate, exploit, and humiliate women by encouraging polygamy, child marriages, and discouraging women from pursuing education. They are alleged to steal adherents from the mainline churches. They also do not have proper worshipping places. Finally, some of them have been accused of performing witch hunting, which results in the dehumanizing of some of their followers.

Despite all these counter allegations, ecumenical dialogue can help both mainline Christians and members of AICs to learn from each other. Both groups are African Christians who believe in the same Triune God, and share the same worldview. Their primary objective is to evangelize Zimbabweans to affect a metanoia. Both read the same scriptures, which they claim to be the inspired word of God. Their humanitarian work complement each other in the communities where they operate. Catholics have hospitals, and AICs have faith healing. Both groups have members who are a mix of sin and grace. Catholics are attempting to implement inculturation, and AICs are already practicing inculturation. When some of the disciples of Jesus complained that they had encountered non-followers who were casting out demons in the name of Jesus and stopped them, Jesus reprimanded them for stopping them, for they were not enemies. Every dialogue needs to be initiated by someone. For any dialogue to succeed, the more powerful should initiate it, and in this case, the mainline churches. They have more resources that may be utilized to facilitate a smooth dialogue. They have the personnel, infrastructure, and a wider worldview when compared to most AICs. That dialogue will benefit them more since their members are being attracted by the AICs.

For any dialogue to be prolific, the parties involved should be convinced that there is a need for such a dialogue. That realization of the need for mutual respect and trust may spring the concerned groups into action. Sincere ecumenical dialogue calls for the equality of the dialoguing partners. There should be a genuine and sincere need to listen and to learn from the other. Dialoguing partners should build on what they agree on, and respect their differences. It would be a noble idea for the mainline churches to establish an apostolate towards AICs, whose mission would be to organize ecumenical workshops, research, talks, and meetings. Such a dialogue will produce mutual understanding of each other, increased trust and respect, borrowing of ideas for the benefit of the people of God, and the eradication of finger-pointing and hatred.

There will be more impediments. Each group thinks that it does not need the other group. The Roman Catholic Church and other mainline churches think that they will not gain anything by pursuing such a dialogue. In fact, some of them boast of their churches that are always full of followers. They are not concerned about the multiple religiosity of some of those followers. Some Catholics lack the humility that is required to pursue ecumenical dialogue because they claim to be more educated, wealthier, and more *civilized*. Some AICs are suspicious of any call for dialogue because they think that its motive is to attack them. There are challenges in pursuing every kind of dialogue, but those who unselfishly commit themselves to understanding and respecting other people in any conversation, will never walk away empty-handed.

10

Women in African Traditional Religion

The issue of the treatment of women in any given religious tradition is controversial, divisive, and debatable. Although such a debate is pertinent, the perspectives of those involved are usually contextual and subjective. They depend on the worldview of the persons who are performing the review. Ordinarily, there are two schools of thought that are involved in such a debate—insiders and outsiders. The outsiders are those people who do not belong to the religion in question, and a few former insiders who have become feminist activists and theologians. Outsiders' views of women in religions other than theirs are sometimes colored by two factors. First, they evaluate the position and treatment of women in other religions in comparison to the treatment of women in their own cultures and religions. Often, they view other religious traditions as oppressive to women. In addition to that, the views of outsiders are sometimes inspired by the idea that "mine is right," and the blatant ignorance of other people's religious traditions.

The second school of thought consists of insiders. This group comprises adherents of a particular religion and a few outsiders who sympathize with the religion in question because of their academic or personal convictions. Despite the demonization of the status of women in a given religion by outsiders, most insiders do not seem to see anything wrong with the way in which they treat their women. In fact, some insiders become defensive whenever the issue of women in their religion is raised. In most cases concerning the position of women in world religions, there are finger-pointing and counter finger-pointing between insiders and outsiders. Since both groups claim that their stance is right, and do have arguments to corroborate it, the best way of exploring the treatment of women in any religious tradition is to look at what both outsiders and insiders say, and the evidence that they provide in support of their views.

The conversation about the position of women in African Traditional Religion has likewise attracted two groups of scholars and adherents. On the one hand, outsiders often argue that African women are oppressed, subjugated, and exploited due to the observation of some religious traditions that are dominated by patriarchal tendencies. On the other hand, insiders usually believe that African women are not oppressed, exploited, and subjugated in any way. Both schools of thought put forward their arguments for upholding the views they have.

Feminist Views

Some African feminist theologians argue that African girls, right from their birth, are socialized to be subordinate to men. Their place is in the home where they help their mothers to do domestic chores and work in the fields, while boys herd cattle and play their games outside. As the girls grow up, they are obliged to be accountable to their fathers and brothers, who guard them more jealously than they do the boys, lest they lose their virginity before marriage. In fact, African boys are left Scot-free, and expected to be more responsible than girls. Of great interest in the upbringing of the Shona girl-child is the preservation of her virginity. The Shona society demands that women should be virgins at marriage. Most African societies have devised ways of shaming the girls who are found to be non-compliant in that respect. Ironically, the same is not demanded of Shona boys, who sometimes brag about the number of virgins they would have deflowered, and the sacred wells from which they would have quenched their thirst, before marriage. In fact, boys are sometimes praised by the society for their premarital sexual exploits. For Mercy Amba Oduyoye, men are double-faced, for they guard their wives and daughters jealously, yet they walk around asking for illicit sexual favors from other men's wives and daughters. For Oduyoye, the demand for a *pure woman* "is solely for the benefit of a man. It has nothing to do with any concern for the woman's physical well-being and very little to do with her spiritual health."[1]

In some countries, the traditional virginity tests have been revived in the guise of protecting women from the HIV/AIDS pandemic. In some parts of South Africa, the girls are graded after their virginity tests, with those who have visible virginity evidence getting the "A" grade, followed by those who are suspected of having had sex once, who get the "B" grade, and the lowest grade being a "C," which is awarded to those women who are believed to have had sex on numerous occasions, and therefore, should be shamed and disgraced.[2] The same virginity tests are not required of men, as if to imply that they are immune to HIV/AIDS infections. Feminist activists see a bias against women there.

1. Oduyoye, "Feminist Theology in an African Perspective," 166–81.
2. Leclerc-Madlala, "Virginity Testing: Managing Sexuality in a Maturing HIV/AIDS Epidemic," 411–22.

The lack of virginity in a woman at marriage can lead her husband to label her as a loose woman, and that can lead to marital complications or even divorce. Carolyn Martin Shaw says that although premarital sex does not prevent a woman from claiming moral superiority, "but if her sexuality and fertility are not claimed by a husband, she can fall into the category of loose woman."[3] One of the most terrible disadvantages of being labeled a *loose woman* is that it becomes extremely hard for such a woman to find a more committed lover. Shona men discuss their prospective wives with their relatives who may discourage them from marrying the so-called *loose women*. The Shona believe that once a woman has shown signs of independence in her sexuality and fertility, then she may never be able to allow any man to exercise any control on her. That woman is considered too independent to marry, and should not be taken seriously in a relationship. Once labelled a loose woman, always a loose woman, goes the fallacious logic. It takes a very brave and a self-differentiated man to marry such a woman. The same label is not applied to men who would have been involved in premarital sex.

In the traditional African society, there were pledging marriages (*kuzvarira*) in which the head of a poor family would pledge one of his little daughters as a future wife to an elderly rich man in exchange for grains and cattle. The little girl is not asked for her opinion, and is deprived of her normal childhood development. As soon as she reached puberty, her husband would snatch her away from her family of origin. She would become a wife and mother at a very tender age. Although most marriages of this nature were successful, some did not last because of the abuse some older men would unleash on their teen wives. Even if the teen wife wished to divorce the older man, it would be difficult for her to find another husband in a society that priced virginity so highly. Her parents would be required to refund the husband, which many poor families could not afford to do. Men were never forced to marry until they were mature and responsible enough to make that decision. Although most Shona people have abandoned pledge marriages, there have been reports of some parents who encourage underage girls to marry older men in some parts of Zimbabwe. Some African Independent Churches have also been accused of this practice.

In the traditional Shona society, a young girl could be used as a compensation wife to pacify avenging spirits. The young woman could be married by one of the brothers of the victim, and the children born out of that wedlock would belong to the *ngozi* spirit. Sometimes, the *ngozi* would not allow its *wife* to get married to any of its relatives. In that case, the woman was supposed to remain single. Sometimes her family would build a special

---

3. Shaw, *Women and Power in Zimbabwe*, 161.

hut for the avenging spirit, and it was the duty of the *ngozi* wife to clean the hut "at regular intervals, to convince it of the family's remembrance."[4] Boys were spared from this practice even if the *ngozi* was a female spirit.

Some African ethnic groups practice clitoridectomy, which refers to the circumcision of women that many states have condemned and outlawed as genital mutilation. This initiation ritual is believed to do more harm than good to the initiates. It can lead to hemorrhage, low sexual drive, infections, and other health complications. It has been argued that female genital mutilation is not intended to benefit women in any way, but men. Patriarchy sells it as a practice that makes women more feminine, modest, and faithful to their husbands, yet men are more concerned with their own selfish needs of keeping women to themselves, even if they cannot satisfy their sexual needs. Although such cultures also circumcise men, the male procedure is not replete with health complications if done under hygienic circumstances. In fact, the circumcision of men is intended for men's well-being rather than the lowering of their sexual libido. Many feminist activists encourage all cultures to abandon the practice of clitoridectomy because it is demeaning and dehumanizing to women. However, this cultural practice is difficult to stamp out, and may continue, clandestinely. Fortunately, in Zimbabwe, there are no cultural groups that perform clitoridectomy to their girls.

The payment of privatized, commercialized, and inflated bridewealth at marriage by Shona men weakens the position of women in the Zimbabwean society. Bridewealth gives more rights to men than to women. The man gets exclusive sexual access to the woman for whom he is paying bridewealth. The same man acquires the rights of ownership over the children born in that marriage.[5] He also gets rights over the productive and reproductive capacities of the women. As if the above rights are not enough, he gets the right to discipline the wife by moderate beating. To worsen the matter, bridewealth is refundable, a situation that might force a woman to stay with an abusive husband because her parents would have used the bridewealth, and cannot refund it. On top of that, the bridewealth negotiations are a preserve of men, and women are barely consulted.[6] Shona children take the totem and the last name of their father. The attainment of these rights by men only, may lead some irresponsible men to abuse their women.

---

4. Daneel, *Old and New in Southern Shona Independent Churches, Vol. 1*, 137.

5. Mukonyora, *Wandering a Gendered Wilderness*, 22.

6. For a detailed explanation of the rights that a man gets after paying bridewealth, read Chitakure, *Shona Women in Zimbabwe—A Purchased People?* 64–78.

When a man dies, his wife is inherited by one of his qualifying relatives. This practice seems to imply that the woman can be treated as part of her husband's property. After the cleansing ceremony, whose purpose is to bring back into the family the spirit of the deceased husband as an ancestor, the widow is supposed to perform the ritual of jumping the weapons (*kudarika vuta*) of her late husband. This ritual is intended to prove that the woman would have been faithful to her late husband in the period between his death and the performance of the cleansing ritual. Any woman who refuses to perform the ritual is suspected of having been unfaithful to her late husband. However, the same ritual is not performed by widowers.

In the traditional Shona society, women could not own land, yet they toiled on the land that belonged to their husbands. Some women would continue to till the land left by their husbands if they remained loyal to the husband's family. This has since changed, although most land owners in Zimbabwe are men. At the traditional courts, women had to be represented by men because they were viewed as equivalent to minors.

One of the biggest imbalances between women and men in Africa concerns polygamy. In most African countries, only men can have as many wives as they can afford. Although polygamy might have served a purpose in the traditional African societies, many feminist theologians think that in most modern African societies, there is no justification for having more than one wife. Polygamy subordinates more women to one man, which makes men feel mightier, prouder, and higher.[7] Some scholars cite the quarrels, jealousy, and fights that polygamous unions experience as sufficient reasons to abandon it. It has been alleged that polygamous men fail to adequately meet the sexual and economical needs of their families. The colonial governments in Africa found the practice of polygamy too archaic and reprehensible as compared to their monogamous culture, and they discouraged it. The missionaries preached that it was the will of God that a man should have one wife, as it was between Adam and Eve, the Christian, Hebrew, and Islamic mythological first couple. African women are not allowed to be polygamous.

In the past, female children could not inherit their father's property, only sons could. Nowadays, the modern law of Zimbabwe does not make any distinction between the male and female child with respect to the inheritance of the deceased's estate, but most Shona people, particularly those who live in the rural areas, exclude daughters when they distribute the estate of their deceased father. This deprivation is made easier by the fact that most women would be married, and living with their husbands. Since the boys

---

7. Nasimiyu-Wasike, "Polygamy: A Feminist Critique," 101–18.

usually live closer to their parents, or even in the same house with them, they easily claim the ownership of the house and other properties. One of the arguments given in support of that deprivation is that if women can benefit from the estate of their deceased father they may enrich the families of their husbands. They would take away the family's wealth and use it for the family of the son-in-law. At the naming ritual that is performed at the end of the cleansing ceremony, the name of the deceased father is inherited by his eldest son even if he is younger than his sisters.

Most of the people who are accused of witchcraft are women. As has been explored in chapter 6 of this book, those accusations are sometimes false and intended to dehumanize the woman, so that whoever abuses her goes unchallenged. A witch is an evil and cannibalistic person who destroys other people's lives by causing misfortunes to happen to them. Mercy Amba Oduyoye observes that a woman can be accused of being a witch for almost everything. If she has more children than other women or is childless, she is a witch; if she is single or widowed, she is a witch; if she is very successful or unsuccessful in a business venture, she is a witch; and if she is quarrelsome, she is a witch, yet men who fall into the same categories are not accused of witchcraft.[8] Once a person is accused of witchcraft, she loses her dignity and support from most people including her own children. The woman accused of witchcraft can be ill-treated without her own relatives and children intervening on her behalf. In the past, those accused of witchcraft could be killed, exiled, or shamed by the whole community. Most of those women would find it difficult to remarry, and consequently die in misery and loneliness. It has been argued that there were power dynamics at play in some of these accusations. Although male witches faced the same punishment, very few men were accused of witchcraft.

In childless marriages, barrenness is almost always blamed on women. A barren woman is disgraced, shamed, and humiliated in the Shona community. She is considered "a dead end and useless to the community."[9] Those women who bore several female children were still found wanting because they did not have male children. African men want to achieve immortality by having many descendants, and any woman who fails to give birth to boys is a threat to that aspiration. In such situations, most men try to resolve the challenge in any way that they deem necessary without the slightest consideration for the need and honor of the women. Some men may marry more wives in their quest for a son. Other men may divorce the woman, and marry another with the expectation of getting a son. Although the determi-

---

8. Oduyoye, *Daughters of Anowa*, 122.
9. Nasimiyu-Wasike, "Polygamy: A Feminist Critique," 101–18.

nation of the sex of a baby is beyond the parents' control, African women are sometimes blamed for the lack of male children, and men are not.

The Conservative View

On the other side, another school of thought argues that African women were not oppressed, exploited, and subjugated in the traditional African society. Isabel Mukonyora emphasizes the point that although African women might have been oppressed, they were never marginalized, "because the domestic domain to which they were central formed the foundation of the public domain."[10] The confinement of African women to the home was to some extent positive. Isabel Mukonyora argues that the Shona home, particularly the round kitchen, which Shona women controlled and managed was the center of power because that is where most religious rituals were celebrated, and political decisions were made. For instance, ancestors were venerated in the kitchen, and bridewealth negotiations were carried out in the same kitchen. For Mukonyora, this was an acknowledgement of the indispensability of the center of the home, the kitchen, and the authority of women.[11] The kitchen has remained the Shona women's sphere of influence up to this day. When sitting in the kitchen, men should follow the kitchen etiquette laid down by women. The kitchen is still the official dinning and sitting room for the rural Shona people. Children are born, nourished, and perhaps die in there. It shows that even ancestors are not threatened by women's presence in the kitchen. So, rather than thinking of the home as a place where women are confined, it is better to view it as a workplace for women, where they take full charge of the management of the home and the family, with the assistance of ancestors, who do not even seem to be afraid of their menstrual blood.

Some people view the requirement of women's virginity as a measure that was intended to protect women rather than to oppress them. It is true that in every society, women are vulnerable to abuse by men in many ways, and most of the time, men can get away with that abuse. One of the worst abuses that women can experience is rape. Rape can be perpetrated by any man, including those that are closely related to the woman. The demand that women be virgins at marriage is likely to have discouraged male relatives from raping their female relatives. Since all of them would be involved in the bridewealth negotiations, and would get something out of the bridewealth, many were compelled to avoid raping their own

10. Mukonyora, *Wandering a Gendered Wilderness*, 24.
11. Ibid., 20.

daughters and sisters because of the shame that would be experienced by the victim at marriage. The requirement of virginity also discouraged men from being involved in premarital sex with the women that they intended to marry. Most men would abstain from premarital sex with the full knowledge that no other man was involved sexually with their girlfriend. More often than not, some men who abstain from premarital sex with their girlfriends are sometimes disappointed when they find out that the wives are not virgins after all the wait. Some men feel that it is disappointing to respect one's girlfriend by abstaining from premarital sex with her, only to discover that somebody would have slept with her. Hence, many men feel that there is no reward for sexual abstinence. A person loses nothing by abstaining from premarital sex, but is likely to lose a lot, if virginity is expected at marriage, but not found.

Those people who carry out virginity tests have also been looked at from a positive side. Usually "women themselves, older and married," are at the forefront of compelling girls to undergo virginity testing.[12] It would be very myopic to view those women as old-fashioned and oppressive to their daughters and granddaughters. Their experiences in life have given them the wisdom that the young women have not yet acquired. What does it profit a woman to lose her virginity to a man who even does not love and care about her, and will probably not dream of marrying her? It is better to preserve one's virginity, and avoid contracting HIV/AIDS than leading a life of sexual indulgence, and then die young. Maintaining one's virginity until marriage can be likened to killing three birds with one stone. First, it prevents the woman from being used by men who do not love her. Second, it protects the woman from contracting sexually transmitted infections. Third, it prevents unwanted pregnancies. Therefore, it has been argued that the requirement for virginity at marriage benefits women too.

What young women need to know is that Shona men are still concerned with virginity, and there is nothing that gives a woman greater pride, authority, control, self-esteem, and freedom, than knowing that her husband found her intact on the first night. The man might not complain about the lack of virginity on the first night, but its absence is an issue that continues to haunt both the wife and the husband all their lives. Some Shona men believe in the saying that goes, *the first cut is the deepest*, and the thought of one being not the perpetrator of that cut makes many men shudder. To encourage young women to keep their virginity is a noble thing, but better methods of imparting that knowledge are needed. Regulations might be put

12. Leclerc-Madlala, "Virginity Testing: Managing Sexuality in a Maturing HIV/AIDS Epidemic," 411–22.

in place to guard against the abusive implementation of any policy, even if it is generally viewed as helpful.

It has also been argued that the female initiation ceremonies prepare girls for childbearing and instruct them on "how to behave as respectable wives and daughters-in-law."[13] These instructions may have contributed to the higher moral standards that African women claim to have, which is a source of their conventional power, and that moral superiority allows them to criticize men before forgiving them, and enables them to draw their sons to their side.[14] Most Shona women believe that *varume imbwa* (men are dogs). This assertion is uttered in comparison between men and women in terms of morality. Initiation ceremonies make African women stronger, more responsible, forgiving, and superior, in terms of morality, and hence, they become qualified to judge men, and condemn those found wanting before forgiving them. That is a lot of power that they wield.

Pledging marriages (*kuzvarira*) violate the rights of children to choose their future marriage partners. However, these pledging marriages were rare despite the presence of abject poverty in the traditional Shona society, because most parents were aware of the human rights violations involved. Every parent who is worth his salts seeks the happiness of his children first and foremost. The parents who pledged their daughters in marriage did that as a last resort to save other children from starvation. In their family of origin, these sacrificed girls were heroes who would have saved their siblings from death. Although most of the pledged girls were too young to consent to the marriage union, some of them lived happy married lives. In fact, some of them were more contented with their marriages than older women who would have chosen their own husbands.

M. F. C. Bourdillon thinks that bridewealth benefits women more than it subjugates them. He claims that it raises their status in their families and societies. The higher the bridewealth received, the greater the woman's status in her family of origin. In fact, a woman's marriage brings more wealth to her family.[15] The traditional bridewealth was intended to safeguard the woman's well-being than oppressing her. All the people who were involved in the bridewealth negotiations wanted the success of the marriage. What has become wrong with bridewealth is the wanton abuse it has suffered because of its privatization and commercialization. If the Shona were to go back to the original bridewealth, most women would feel more protected and less vulnerable.

13. Thomas, *Politics of the Womb*, 15.
14. Shaw, *Women and Power in Zimbabwe*, 127.
15. Bourdillon, *The Shona Peoples*, 50.

The inheritance of a widow by one of the qualifying members of her late husband's family was intended to cushion the widow and her children from the harsh conditions that resulted from the loss of the sole breadwinner. The Shona knew how difficult it was for widows to take the position of both mother and father in the family. They also knew that it would be very difficult for a widow to get a new husband if she were older. Consequently, her inheritance was intended to provide her with a husband and livelihood. No woman was forced to choose to be inherited as a wife. Most inherited women continued to live in their marital homes, managing the family with the help of the new husband, who would visit them occasionally, if he already had a family of his own.

Polygamy has been cited as one of the traditional practices that oppressed African women. Although most feminist theologians have looked at it from a political and economic point of view, polygamy is also caused by religious beliefs that both African men and women uphold as sacrosanct. In some cases, polygamy is a result of a belief that women are not ritually clean during menstrual periods, and after the birth of a child. During these times, sex is forbidden. In some African societies, sexual activities were forbidden when a woman reached menopause. Some men married more than one wife to cater for their sexual needs during those times when they could not be intimate with their wives. Some wives were inherited as a way to take care of their economic and sexual needs. Polygamy is also said to have been permitted to enable excess women to have husbands. Men died in wars and during hunting errands, and thus, some societies had more women than men. It has been argued that the societies, which unwaveringly uphold monogamy, do sometimes practice concubinage, which is a worse form of polygyny because such women are never recognized as official wives of the men that use them. In African polygamous unions, the wives and children have the protection and support of the husband and father, respectively. In fact, in Zimbabwe, the abandonment of polygamy has ushered in a new polygamous union called small-housing (mistresses), which makes both the women involved and their children vulnerable to all sorts of abuse.[16] However, I do not intend to portray polygamy as a marriage institution that is perfect because there is no form of marriage that is perfect.

It has been argued that senior African women could participate in the preparation of rituals, and some of them presided over the celebration of some rituals. The spirit of Ambuya Nehanda became the inspiration to the people of Zimbabwe during the second Chimurenga because of her heroic defense of the Shona people's territorial integrity and national sovereignty

---

16. Chitakure, *Shona Women in Zimbabwe—A Purchased People?* 52–55.

during the First War of Liberation (*Chimurenga*) (1896–98). Isabel Mukonyora highlights the importance of the sacred storytelling (*ngano*) that traditional Shona women employed to teach African philosophy.[17] Women are also privileged to be *ambuya nyamukutas* (midwives), who facilitate the perpetuity of humanity.

Summing up

Having surveyed what both schools of thought say about the position of African women in society and religion, the verdict depends on the worldview of the judge. Some people still think that there is more that needs to be done to emancipate African women from the dominance of patriarchal systems. There are religious practices that subjugate women, such as child marriage, avenging spirits wives, clitoridectomy, the blame of women for barrenness, deprivation of female children to inherit their father's estate, accusation of witchcraft, and other practices that should not be defended by anyone who respects women. It is interesting to note that some of the defenders of religious and cultural practices that are believed to oppress women are women themselves. They see nothing wrong with those practices, and they claim to be the insiders who have experienced those things.

African Women, Modernity, and Christianity

The encounter between African women and the European culture has had an impact upon the position of African women in African societies. The introduction of European education brought both boys and girls into the same classroom, studying the same disciplines. Most African women had an opportunity to prove that they were as intelligent as men, and in some cases, more intelligent than men. Although women were initially left alone to manage rural homes, families, and farming when their husbands went to work in the newly established factories, mines, and farms, they managed to produce enough food to sustain their families. When they were awarded the opportunity to work alongside their male counterparts in towns, they proved that they were as good as men, and probably better.

In many African countries, women serve in the public and private sectors, and they continue to shine alongside their male counterparts. The introduction of equal educational opportunities encouraged African women to showcase their talents and wisdom. Although in most African cultures,

---

17. Mukonyora, *Wandering the Gendered Wilderness*, 32.

women who are gainfully employed are still expected to perform the traditional chores and tasks when they come back from work, most have proved that they can stoically wear the two hats of being bosses at their workplaces, and mothers and wives at their homes.

Most Christian churches in Africa tried to bring women to par with men, but they encountered many challenges. Some churches challenged witchcraft beliefs that almost always condemned more women as witches than men. They challenged polygamy, which allowed men to marry as many wives as they wanted. However, the way the Christian churches attempted it ended up harming the women themselves. The Roman Catholic Church allowed the man to remain with only one wife by divorcing the rest, which caused a lot of suffering to the divorced women. The Roman Catholic Church did not encourage polygamous men to do that for the sake of liberating women, but for the liberation of men from evil cultural practices. It seems it was up to the converted polygamous men either to keep his wives or be expelled from the RCC. There is no evidence that the affected women were consulted about their ordeal. Of course, the missionaries advised the converted polygamous men to continue to support their affected wives, but the RCC had no police force to oblige the men to support the expelled wives.

One of the challenges that the Christian churches continue to face in Africa is the dominance of patriarchy. Christianity was founded by Jesus Christ, a Jew, who was born in a culture where women were not viewed as equal to men. In the New Testament, some biblical passages command women to respect their husbands but not commanding the men to do the same, and by so doing, encouraging inequality within the church. In addition, Jesus himself did not choose any woman to be one of his twelve apostles, an argument that the Roman Catholic Church uses to deny ordination to Catholic women. Although that rule may seem unfair, the fact is that it is based on the Bible. The RCC thus considers itself to be faithful to the scriptures. Moreover, both men and women have the same religious obligations in many Christian churches, but in most cases, men are the leaders of the church. Furthermore, those women who refused to be spiritual subordinates to men and started their own churches, in Zimbabwe, such as Mai Chaza of the Guta raJehova (City of God), were scorned at by the mainline churches.

Of course, Christianity can be credited for bringing women and men in the same church, worshipping God side by side, but it seems that women have remained inferior to men, even in the house of God. Mercy Amba Oduyoye feels that "The African Church needs to empower women not to speak for themselves and manage their 'women's affairs', but to be fully present in decisions and operations that affect the whole church, including the forming of its theology."[18] Some Protestant churches have made great strides in empowering women in their churches, but the dream of women becoming leaders of the Roman Catholic Church seems to be a wild goose chase. Recently, Pope Francis has allowed some research into the RCC's traditions concerning the ordination of women to the diaconate—a good sign.

Some African Independent Churches subject their female followers to more oppression and segregation than mainline churches. Some encourage polygamy and child marriages in which young girls are given away in marriage to older church members. Some prevent women from accessing modern reproductive health medicines, and by so doing, preventing women from taking charge of family planning and their own health. As if that is not bad enough, some AICs forbid menstruating women from entering the sacred spaces where worship takes place, and that deprives women of the graces that emanate from the communal worship of God. It also embarrasses the woman who is prevented from entering the holy place because every church member would know that she is having her monthly periods. Mercy Amba Oduyoye argues that "The church must shed its image as a male organization with a female clientele whom it placates with vain promises, half truths, and the prospect of redemption at the end of time."[19]

---

18. Oduyoye, *Beads and Strands*, 97.
19. Oduyoye, *Daughters of Anowa*, 185.

11

Shona Ethics

Good character and acceptable behavior are crucial in Shona morality because every person is expected to possess them. The Shona refer to good character and behavior as *unhu*, which should be the essence of every human being. The word *unhu* comes from the Shona noun, *munhu* that means a human being. *Unhu* differentiates a person from other animals. It includes virtues such as integrity, honest, trustworthiness, reliability, responsibility, respect, among others. One is considered a human being because he possesses *unhu*—the humanness of a person. *Unhu* can be used interchangeably with the word *tsika*, which means behavior. The Shona may refer to a person who lacks *unhu* as a dog (*imbwa*), meaning that the person in question would have lost the essence of being human, and would have assumed the essence of a cold-blooded brute. When the Shona describe a person as *haana unhu*, they mean that he has a bad character or behavior. A person who lacks *unhu* is untrustworthy, unreliable, dishonest, irresponsible, disrespectful, arrogant, and has no integrity. In other words, he lacks the essence of being human, and therefore, may not be fit to be called a person. The Shona evaluate one's *unhu* or lack of it through the way one carries himself about, and how he relates to others.

Greetings

One of the most crucial aspects of *unhu* is the respect that one renders to oneself and others. This respect or lack of it, manifests in many different areas of the Shona relationships. Appropriate greetings are crucial in the Shona morality. Every greeting should be appropriate to the age, gender, relationship, and familiarity between the persons involved. Most greetings may indicate the time of the day at which they are being exchanged. Generally, the younger persons are expected to initiate the greetings. The greeting for the morning is *mangwanani*, which means good morning. The response is *mangwanani*. This greeting is immediately followed by, *mamuka sei* or *marara sei* (did you wake up well or did you sleep well?). The response is, *tamuka kana mamamukawo*, or *tarara kana mararawo* (we woke up well if you also woke up well, or we slept well if you also slept well), to which the inquirer must answer, *tamuka* or *tarara* (we woke up well, we slept well). This greeting is for people who live in the same home and neighborhood, particularly those who would have seen each other within a couple of days. Even those people who sleep in the same room are expected to exchange these greetings as soon as they wake up.

If it is after midday, the greeting is *masikati* (good afternoon). The response is the same, *masikati*. *Masikati* is immediately followed by *maswera sei* (how was your day?). The response to that greeting is *taswera kana maswerawo* (It was a good day if your day was also good). If it is at night, the greeting is *manheru* or *madekwani* (good evening). The response is *manheru* or *madekwani*. The inquirer then asks, *maswera sei*, and the response is, *taswera kana maswerawo*.

If the people greeting each other would have not seen each other for a while, say about three days or more; the greeting is different, especially the second part. Instead of saying *mangwanani*, the inquirer says, *mhoroi* or *kwaziwai*. This greeting is sometimes accompanied by the hand shake if the persons are within each other's reach, and are not prohibited from shaking hands, by the nature of their relationship. The response is *mhoroi* or *kwaziwai*. The inquirer then says, *makadini* (how are you?) The response to that should be, *tiripo, makadiniwo* (we are alright, and, how are you?)

Although either of the persons involved in any greeting may take the initiative, it is always the junior who should initiate the second half of the greeting. But, there are exceptions to this rule. All nephews and nieces, even if they are older than their uncles or aunts, should initiate the inquiry about the other person's health. The son-in-law is considered a junior to his father-in-law, mother-in-law, and brothers-in-law. Young brothers inquire about the health of older brothers. Some Shona groups require all sisters to initiate the second part of the greetings when interacting with their brothers. Seniority in terms of age and relationship is crucial. Some people may first confirm their ages and relationship before they inquire about each other's health.

It is also important to remember that the greetings should be exchanged when people are sitting, kneeling, or standing depending on their relationship and ages. Sometimes the son-in-law should kneel when greeting the mother-in-law. The greetings should be accompanied by some rhythmic clapping of the hands (*kuombera/kuuchira*). If the relationship between the inquirer and the one who is responding is known by those involved, the relationship title should be used in the greeting. For instance, children should always say, *mamuka sei amai* or *baba* (did you sleep well, mom, or dad?). The Shona address women of their mother's age in the same way they address their biological mothers unless they are related otherwise. All men of their father's age may be addressed as *father* unless the involved people are related otherwise. Young women may be addressed as *sisters*, and young men as *brothers*, even if they are strangers.

Usually, there are pauses between each set of greeting. It is also interesting to note that the greeting is in the plural form, not singular. The reason for using the plural is that the greeting is intended for the persons who are involved, and also their family members who might be at home. Although some inquirers will also ask about the welfare of others in general, the one responding to any greeting is supposed to include them. She might tell the enquirer about those who are not feeling well, if any.

The response to the second part of the Shona greetings, *tamuka kana mamukawo* (we woke up well if you also did the same), *taswera kana maswerawo* (our day was good if yours was also good), *tinofara kana muchifarawo* (we are well if you too are well), are crucial to *unhu* philosophy. These responses exhibit the heart of *unhu*, for they show the interdependence and connectedness of the Shona people. One cannot claim to be in good health if her neighbor or relative is sick, or has experienced a misfortune of any kind. Anything that bothers one member of the community is also of concern to the other person. If one person is sick, the whole village is affected. If one villager is hungry, it becomes the responsibility of those who know about it to feed him. *Unhu* dictates that no one should suffer alone because the joys, sorrows, and tribulations of life should be shared by the community. The Shona greetings may take longer, but the listeners will always act upon what they are told in those greetings. That is what it means to be *munhu* (human being). Once they get to know of the ill-health of one of the villagers, the neighbors are expected to visit him. They too should empathize with those who would have lost a family member.

The first sign of one's possession of humanness is seen in the way one greets others. Any person who does not greet other people, and inquire about their health is a social misfit and has no *unhu*. Refusal to return greetings is considered a disgrace and an insult. A person who repeatedly refuses to return greetings is suspected of being a witch. It is every person's responsibility to greet others, listen to their challenges, and do something about it. The Shona greet each other, and spend some time listening to each other because they believe that it is their duty to help their neighbors if necessary.

Filial and Fraternal Respect

One's *unhu* is also assessed through one's interactions with relatives. The Shona have an intricate network of relationships, which determine the nature of one's behavior in the presence of such people. One's parents should be treated with utmost respect. Children should enquire about their parents' health every day, or whenever they can. They are expected to respect them in any manner possible. Grandparents should be accorded more respect because they are the progenitors of the family. One should also respect one's older brothers and sisters. In the Shona culture, the term brother refers to one's blood brothers and all the sons of one's uncles (his father's brothers). The daughters of one's uncles are also one's sisters. There are no cousins in the Shona relationship networks. When eating together, the oldest brother should be the first to take a lump or spoon of food, followed by the second oldest, in descending older. The younger brothers refer to the older brother as *babamukuru* (senior father). Usually, the oldest son inherits the name of the father after his death, and he is expected to assume the authority of his late father thereafter. Nephews should respect uncles. It must be noted that the respect is always reciprocal.

The most significant relationship is between the son-in-law *(mukwasha)* and mother-in-law *(amai),* or sister-in-law (wife of wife's brother) *(ambuya).* The *mukwasha* pays a small fee to get the initial permission to greet his *ambuya*. There should not be any shaking of hands between the duo. Both *mukwasha* and *ambuya* should kneel, facing opposite directions when greeting each other. Both should clap hands as they greet each other. Ordinarily, *mukwasha* and *ambuya* should not sit in the same room. When *mukwasha* visits the in-laws, he is accommodated in his own room where he can be entertained by the sisters of his wife *(varamu)*. These sisters are considered to be his future wives, if any situation arises that requires his father-in-law to offer him another wife. Some *vakwasha* take advantage of this relationship and end up abusing their *varamu*. In the past, *mukwasha* was allowed to tease his *muramu* in any way, but he was not expected to be intimate with her. Some wives raise their young sisters, and their husbands are expected to respect them. A *mukawasha* whose virgin *muramu* gets married to another man while under his care, should receive a small token of appreciation *(sukamachende)* from the husband. *Sukamachende* literally means, the cleansing of the testicles of the *mukwasha,* and is offered to the *mukwasha* by a junior *mukwasha* via the father-in-law, for having respected, and not violated the *muramu* before marriage. So, the kind of respect given to people depends on the relationship between the people involved. A person who does not show appropriate respect to other people is deficient in *unhu*.

The Shona avoid calling adults by their first names, if they are married, or if they have children. Once a woman is married, she ceases to be called by her maiden names. Before she has her first child, her totem or sub-totem is used as her name. For instance, if her totem is *gumbo* (cow's leg), she becomes Magumbo. If she belongs to the lion (*shumba*) totem, she becomes Masibanda. If she belongs to the heart totem (*moyo*), she becomes Mamoyo. The totem name is the greatest honor given to a married woman before she bears her first child. This title may continue to be used for her together with other titles and names until her death. Once she gives birth to her first born, the woman assumes the name of her child. If the firstborn child is Nyasha, she becomes Mai Nyasha (mother of Nyasha). Although the totem name still holds, the firstborn child's name is more popular among the Shona. Even the woman's own parents and siblings address her using her firstborn's name. Calling a married woman by her first name is a sign of disrespect and lacks of *unhu*. The woman might be your friend, sister, or niece, but once she gets married, she deserves to be respected. Her maiden names may remain on her official documents, and may only be used when engaging in official business transactions that require official names.

Eventually, the married woman may assume a third name, which is her husband's family name. If she is married to Chitakure, she becomes Mai Chitakure (mother of Chitakure). In the past, this name would be merited through the length of the period of one's marriage. Usually, the name of the family was reserved for the mother-in-law (husband's mother). However, the family name can be used even by newly married women if they are working as teachers, nurses, and other occupations in which such names are used officially. It is very rare to know the official names of women in the Shona neighborhood, unless they were born there. Calling a married woman by her maiden names in non-official situations exhibits the lack of *unhu* in the person who does that.

The same applies to a married man. Before he has a child, his in-laws may call him by his sub-totem. For instance, if his totem is cow leg (*gumbo*), he becomes Madyirapazhe. If the totem is shumba Sigauke (lion), he is referred to as Sigauke. However, the man's family members may continue to call him by his first name, and that is not considered disrespectful. Once the couple has their first child, the man too is called by the name of his firstborn. For instance, if the child is Mufaro, he becomes Baba Mufaro (father of Mufaro). Eventually, he may be called by his family name, which up to a certain period, is reserved for his father, uncles, and grandfather, if alive.

Calling adults by their first names shows that one is wanting regarding *unhu*. Close family members may occasionally use the first name of a married woman as a sign of endearment. However, if it is overdone, it might be interpreted as disrespectful. This requirement is also observed by married couples, who should stop using each other's first name as soon as they get married. If they continue to use each other's first names, they would be considered disrespectful to each other, and to those around them. They may use their firstborn's name or sub-totem for each other. In addition to that, married men and women may refer to each other as *mother* or *father* respectively. Usually, the two get into the habit of calling each other *mother* or *father* during their children's socialization. The firstborn must be taught that the man in the house is his father by imitating his mother, and the same applies to the mother.

As they grow up, boys and girls are socialized differently. Boys and girls play different games and spend most of their time in different places. In the past, boys would herd the cows, hunt, and play soccer. Girls' sphere of influence was the kitchen where they learnt how to cook, wash dishes and clothes, and take care of their siblings. Of course, there were also games in which both boys and girls participated. The Shona children are taught to respect their own and other people's bodies. Premarital sex is prohibited, although girls are held more accountable if they lose virginity before marriage. In the past, girls that were found to have lost their virginity before marriage were shamed and demeaned. However, the premarital loss of virginity was not a major cause for divorce. This requirement does not mean that single mothers are not respected and cannot find marriage partners—they do. Many Shona men demand openness from the woman who they intend to marry. Those women who do not reveal their single-mother status to their would-be husbands may encounter challenges in the future when the husbands become aware of the secrets. Most Shona groups do not emphasize or require the virginity of boys at all. However, engaging in premarital sex by boys is considered lack of *unhu*.

Sexual Integrity

Sex talk is only allowed between same-sex friends. Parents, siblings, and strangers may not talk about sex explicitly. The Shona rarely use the proper names of the sexual organs when talking to their children. Even those people who are permitted to talk about sex use symbolic names for the organs. For instance, the penis might be referred to as the cooking stick, the vagina, as the well, the sexual act, as cooking, and so on. Each locality has its sexual euphemism. In each village, there are some people who lack *unhu*, who may use sexual implicit language (*kuwonyoka/kutsveruka*). Kissing in public is not allowed, even if it is between married couples. Parents do not kiss each other in the presence of their children because *hazvina unhu* (it lacks *unhu*). Hugs between relatives are rarely given in public. Even married people avoid hugging each other in public. This avoidance of public show of intimacy does not mean that Shona husbands do not love their wives—they do, perhaps more than those people who publicly show their affection. The parents' bedroom is a no-go area for adult children unless they have been asked to perform a task therein. The parents' bedroom is sacred space. A person who uses explicit sexual language is considered wanting in terms of *unhu*.

Sexual misconduct is a result of lack of *unhu*. There are three sexual misconducts that the Shona take seriously. First, incest is a pernicious offence that does not only offend the living family members of the perpetrator, but also the ancestors and God. In the past, if anyone committed incest, he would be banished from the clan forever. The ancestors would be so offended that they would temporarily withdraw rain from the whole community, and both animals and people would suffer because of that. A ritual had to be performed to appease the offended spirits. One should never have any sexual activity with one's brothers, sisters, parents, cousins, nieces, nephews, aunts, and many others. The prohibition is even stricter between sons-in-law, mothers-in-law, and sisters-in-law (wife's, brother's wife). They should not touch each other's hands when greeting. They should not be left alone in the same room if it can be avoided. For the Shona, incest is the worst sexual misconduct one can ever commit.

The other sexual misconduct is adultery in which one or both partners are married. If the two are apprehended, the illicit lover should pay compensation to the formal husband. Traditionally, the compensation was determined by the village head or the chief's court. However, no man was persuaded to continue living with an adulterous woman if he wanted to divorce her. Both the man and woman who are involved in such an affair are criticized for having no *unhu*. Lawful sexual activity is between married people and should be performed secretly, in their bedroom. The Shona official time for sex is the night, when all the children and people who might overhear the noise are asleep. In the traditional Shona homestead, the minimization of sexual noises was easy because they had separate round huts that were positioned away from each other. The long distance between bedrooms was intended to eliminate the noise that could come out of the sacred activity. No one, except the couple should know what they do in their bedroom. The only evidence that the Shona children have concerning their parents' sexual life, is their existence. Those Shona people who do not conceal their sexual activities are deficient in *unhu*.

The third sexual misconduct is rape case (*chibharo*), and is detested by the Shona people. Men are not allowed to force women to have sex with them. Only adult men and women who are in love may have sex, if both consent to it. Traditionally, it was believed that no unmarried woman with *unhu* would agree to have sex with her boyfriend, even if she wanted to do it. Consequently, some men used some level of persuasive force to which the woman would respond affirmatively or negatively. It was believed that if the woman did not want to have sex, she would let the boyfriend know in no uncertain terms. In cases like that, any reasonable man was expected to respect the wishes of the woman. Women had to be very careful if they did not want to be involved in premarital sex. For instance, they were to avoid seeing their boyfriends in secluded places, at night, and in the boyfriends' bedrooms. Although many men respected the wishes of their women, some found it difficult to tell if the woman's preliminary refusal to having sex was just customary, or serious. They had to watch the woman carefully and closely to identify any signs of her interest in having sex. If it was discovered that a man had forced himself upon a woman or had consensual sex, the parents of the woman could chase her away from home so that she eloped with the culprit.

Nowadays, Shona parents instruct their children to stay away from premarital sex. Anyone who forces himself upon another person sexually can be arrested for that. Raping women (*kubhinya*) is a sign of moral bankruptcy. It is one of the most shameful criminal offenses in Zimbabwe. There have been cases where women have also raped men, and the shame attached to that crime is even worse. One of the biggest challenges that the Shona have been experiencing is the embarrassment attached to reporting rapists that are related to the victims. This avoidance is largely caused by the taboo against incest. Some families do not want the public to know that their daughter was raped by a relative because of the shame and embarrassment caused to both the survivor and the perpetrator. Also, the Shona do not talk about marital rape because of the reasons explored in chapter 2.

The Dress Code

The Shona are concerned about how a person dresses since they believe that one's *unhu* may be mirrored by one's dressing. Mini-skirts and short dresses are not encouraged, as they are associated with the lack of *unhu*. Some Shona people criticize the wearing of trousers or pants by women, since they are likely to reveal the shapes of their bodies. However, in most urban areas, many Shona people have accepted mini-skirts and pants (trousers) as acceptable and decent dressing for women. It has been argued that there is no connection between one's moral aptitude and her way of dressing. It should be noted that in the rural areas most elders have not accepted mini-skirts and trousers/pants as normal dressing for women. Those women who feel comfortable in pants or mini-skirts in urban areas, may not feel at ease to wear them in their rural homes, in the presence of their brothers and fathers. Dressing inappropriately can be interpreted as a sign of one's deficiency in *unhu*. A woman with *unhu* is expected to wear appropriate dresses at appropriate times, and in appropriate places. If a woman thinks that her dress is too short for some elders' comfort, she should wrap up her dresses with a blanket or piece of cloth named *zambia*, to cover a good portion of their legs.

The dress code is not as strict for Shona men as it is for women. Men can wear shorts or stay shirtless, and are still considered decently and appropriately dressed. Of course, Zimbabwean men have been affected by fashion trends from the West. Most Shona parents and elders do not approve of the sagging pants/trousers that some young men seem to be fond of. The boys who dress like that are considered deficient as far as *unhu* is concerned. Tattoos and earrings worn by men are also not well-received by the Shona elders, and the men who have them are believed to be wanting in terms of *unhu*.

Thou Shalt Not Steal and Kill

The Shona teach their children to respect private property by avoiding stealing. If one wants something that her neighbor or relative has, she should ask for it rather than steal it. The other ethical code concerns killing, which is forbidden for any reason. Human life is sacred, and should never be taken away for any reason. Before the coming of Western jails to Zimbabwe, murderers were asked to pay compensation to the family of the victims. If the perpetrator was not apprehended, the avenging spirit of the victim would haunt the perpetrator's family until reparations were paid. Nowadays, the Shona punish murderers twice. First, they may be sent to jail if found guilty of the offence by the criminal courts of the country. Second, their families may be required to pay compensation to appease the avenging spirit of the victim. If the offender is acquitted by a criminal court because of any reason, he may still pay compensation to the family of the dead person. The payment of compensation has nothing to do with the criminal justice system of the country, but is enforced by the avenging spirit of the wronged as has been explored in chapter 5.

Gratitude

Gratitude is encouraged right from childhood. Children are taught to clap their hands as a symbol of gratitude whenever they receive a gift, and before and after eating any food. The mother or the giver may withdraw the gift or food if the receiver does not clap his hands as a sign of appreciation. Just clapping one's hands is considered a sufficient show of one's thankfulness. Nowadays, many parents teach their children to say, "thank you" (*tatenda*), in addition to clapping. The Shona have a proverb, which goes, "*kusatenda uroyi*," which can be translated as, failure to thank someone is as bad as witchcraft. Ingratitude is like witchcraft because it destroys the giver's love, which would have driven her to offer the gift.

The traditional Shona women are expected to kneel when thanking someone. Usually they recite the totemic poem of the person they are thanking. Shona children are encouraged to use both hands when receiving a gift even if it is small. If the situation requires the use of one hand, the right hand is preferred. It is considered lack of *unhu* to receive a gift or greet elders using the left hand even if one is left handed. The gratitude should appear to be sincere and coming from one's heart. Children are also encouraged to learn to exchange gifts to fulfill the proverb, "*kandiro kanoenda kunobva kamwe*," which calls for the reciprocation of gifts. After consuming one's food, one is expected to clap hands as a sign of his thankfulness. Showing one's gratitude is a must among the Shona, and failure to do so is a sign of the lack of *unhu*. Although, the Shona talk of *kutenda kwekitsi kuri mumoyo* (The gratitude of a cat is internal or in its heart), it is discouraged not to show one's thankfulness openly.

Generosity

Generosity is expected of every Shona person. One should always be ready to share whatever one has with those who do not have. No one should be denied food if he needs it. In fact, Shona people offer food to strangers and neighbors even if they do not need it. Food should be shared, and it is an insult to refuse to accept hospitality. A visitor is not asked if she needs food or not because that is considered a sign of selfishness. Food should be offered without asking the visitor if he needs it or not. During times of drought when food is scarce, the Shona share the little that they do have with those who are starving. When one is travelling, and it is about to rain, one may ask for shelter from any nearest home, and the owner is obliged to offer the sojourner temporary accommodation. If the night comes and one has not yet reached his destination, she may ask for overnight shelter from any homeowner close by. The villagers who do have cars may offer transport for free to those who do not have. The owners may accept a token of gratitude in the form of money, but what pushes them to assist is their concern for others. Those with bicycles do not deny the use of such property to those who do not have.

It is very interesting to note that the Shona do not readily and explicitly accept the gratitude that is verbally offered to them. When someone says, "*Tatenda*" (thank you), the Shona respond by saying, "*Muchitendei*" (don't thank me). This response shows the giver's sense of duty and humility. The Shona do not have the phrase for, "You are welcome" as a response to "Thank you." The refusal to accept the verbal gratitude comes from the belief that each person is responsible for taking care of another person, even if they are not related. It is one's responsibility to offer food to the hungry, water to the thirsty, and clothes to the naked. One is expected to offer hospitality without expecting anything in return.

Non-Violence

Shona children are taught to be peaceful in settling disputes, and the use of violence is discouraged. Although men were allowed to discipline their wives by moderate beating, the abuse of one's wife was condemned by almost everybody. Fighting is allowed as the last resort, and never as the only way of resolving issues. Children are strongly instructed not to engage in fighting at school. If two people are seen fighting in public, the first impulse of bystanders is to pacify them. Fighting is for brutes, not rational human beings.

Unhu sums up the way a Shona person should live. It is believed that *unhu* can be learnt from one's parents. Therefore, the lack of *unhu* is sometimes blamed on the parents.[1] Consequently, the lack of *unhu* in one's children embarrasses the parents. If the parents lack *unhu*, it may be assumed that their children are also deficient in *unhu*. In this case, children may pay for the sins of their parents. *Unhu* is what young men and women look for when hunting for a marriage partner. A woman may marry a very rich man, but if he has no *unhu* that marriage may not stand the test of time. A man can possess the world, but without *unhu*, he is just like a wild animal. A woman might be as beautiful as an angel, but without *unhu*, her

---

1. Gelfand, "UNHU: The Personality of the Shona."

beauty is worthless. Men look for a woman of character and integrity, not just outward looks or earthly possessions. Misfortune may take away one's beauty, wealth, and some body organs, but if that person clings to *unhu*, he is better off than a thousand men who lack *unhu*.

Shona Ethics and Christianity

The introduction of urbanization and Christianity in Zimbabwe had both positive and adverse consequences on the Shona way of life. The Shona way of greeting has suffered a major setback because of urbanization and industrialization. In urban areas, people have become so busy that they scarcely have enough time to greet every person that they meet in public transportation and along the streets. People in town are ruled by the *chronos* time, which dictates that they be at their work places not later than some specified time. When they finish work, they are in a rash to get transport back to their homes. There is no enough time to inquire about other people's well-being on those busy streets.

The other challenge concerns the cultural diversity of the people who live in towns. Unlike in the rural setting, where everyone knows almost everyone, in towns, people come from all over the country, and are sometimes complete strangers, who may feel that they have no obligation to greet their neighbors. The nature of town life demands that people mind their own business, and should interact with their relatives. The people who migrate to urban areas find it disturbing and disillusioning that town folks do not have the courtesy to stop and greet each other. Churches have bridged the gap by becoming places where people can relate and greet each other the way they are used to do in the rural areas. On Sundays and other prayer days, the people who yearn for the rural *unhu* get a glimpse and feel of the old golden days.

The other challenge that the Shona have encountered because of the modernization of the society concerns relationships. Some of the people who live in towns rarely visit their rural homes, and that leads to their offspring losing touch with the rural life, traditional ethical codes, and relatives. In addition to that, some relatives who live in towns no longer visit each other as much as they used to do due to the scarcity of resources, accommodation, and the spirit of individualism that has gripped them. Relatives who used to be the teachers of morality are now thinly spread out in distant cities of the country, and that makes it difficult for frequent visits. Now, with the elders living far away in the rural areas, and the uncles and aunts in different cities, the Shona youth have been deprived of the traditional teachers of Shona ethics.

The accommodation challenges in towns lead parents and children to sleep in rooms next to each other, or sometimes, in the same bedroom, which violates the privacy that should be maintained between parents and their children. The relationship between the son-in-law and mother-in-law has also been affected. When *ambuya* or *mukwasha* visits each other in towns, the accommodation situation forces them to live in the same house, and sit in the same room, which is a scandal to the rural folk. In some cases, the accommodation challenges in urban areas have led to the commission of incest. However, this point does not minimize the incest that can also be committed in rural areas. To a greater extent, the church has contributed in bringing people under one roof irrespective of their relationships. But most churches have maintained the traditional gender separation during worship by seating men and women separately. The Christian churches have provided teachers of morality to fill in the gap that has been left by the traditional elders.

One of the most embarrassing violation of the Shona ethical code happens at church weddings when the presiding officer asks the bridegroom to kiss the bride. Most couples comply although it is taboo to kiss one's wife in the presence of other people. It is considered lack of *unhu* to show that kind of intimacy in the company of the mother-in-law, father-in-law, and other relatives (*vanyarikani*). The traditional Shona elders may feel embarrassed by the public kissing of one's bride, for it lacks *unhu*. A man with *unhu* does not kiss his wife in public, but since people respect the pastor and the laws of their church, they do comply to perform that shameful sacrifice. The Christian churches and the civil society discourage the *chiramu* relationships that may lead to intimacy. Although there are still Shona people who tease each other as *varamu*, they respect the boundaries—no intimacy.

The other aspect of the Shona ethics that continues to encounter challenges is the use of first names for women, which has been interpreted both negatively and positively. Some people argue that calling married women by their first names is a violation of the Shona moral code, and is disrespectful to them. On the other hand, other people have interpreted it as part of the empowerment of the Shona women. The missionaries went a step further in bridging the gap between boys and girls by encouraging both to receive the same type of education. Unlike in the traditional rural home, where boys and girls played separately, the Western education brought them together in the same classroom where they learn as equals. Some Christian churches such as the Roman Catholic Church have maintained that men and women are equal though different.

Although the traditional Shona society tried to enforce a higher level of morality, some sexual misconduct could go unpunished. In cases of rape, the perpetrator could get away with it if he agrees to marry the victim or pay compensation, which may have been traumatizing to the woman. In the past, incest could be swept under the carpet to save the face of the offender and to cushion the survivor from shame. The modern justice system ensures that perpetrators of sexual misconduct are sent to jail for a very long time. Although some Christian leaders have been found wanting in that area, most of them support and uphold the criminal laws of the country.

The dress code has been a subject of debate in the Shona society. The Christian churches and the traditional culture agree that people should dress decently in church and at home. Some churches forbid women to wear pants/trousers and mini-dresses to church. Some Roman Catholic parishes demand that all women put on veils before receiving Holy Communion as a sign of reverence. Consequently, most Christian guilds have established uniforms that their followers wear to church. Men too are expected to dress decently. Shorts are not allowed in churches, although some men may get away with tight fitting trousers. Some work places have dress codes too. Most primary and secondary schools in Zimbabwe require their students to wear uniforms. In most cases, girls wear dresses and boys, trousers. However, there are schools that do allow female students to wear trousers. The Christian churches and the traditional Shona society seem to enforce the same type of *unhu* in terms of the dress code.

The church and the Shona society agree on their teachings concerning stealing and killing. The Shona teaches that if a person kills another person, he should be arrested and pay compensation to the family of the victim. If compensation is not paid, then, the spirit of the victim would come back to demand justice by punishing the family of the perpetrator. Christian churches view the same issue differently. They teach that murderers should be sent to jail, and if they do not repent, they will eventually go to hell. If murderers confess their sins, they should still go to jail, but may still go to heaven. The Shona do not believe in forgiveness without reparations, for they believe that true reconciliation is not cheap—one pays for it. Moreover, the traditional Shona do not have the concept of hell because the spirit of the wronged can punish the wrongdoers.

Both the Christian churches and the traditional Shona agree on the requirement of sexual morality for both single and married people. Although Christian churches do not stress the need for premarital virginity, some Shona people still take that seriously. Both encourage marital faithfulness and condemn infidelity of either partner. However, Shona people allow divorce if the woman is unfaithful, but for the Roman Catholic Church, infidelity of either party does not render a consummated and ratified marriage dissoluble. The Shona allow polygamy, but most churches condemn it.

Therefore, it seems that the encounter between Christianity and the Shona culture has benefitted and affected the latter. There are areas of agreement and disagreement. Most Shona Christians, particularly those who tap from both religious traditions, have benefitted more. They have produced an ethical code that derives from both the Christian and traditional ethical codes. Where Christianity seems to be lacking, they turn to their traditional ways of doing things, and the other way around. However, some Shona people have come to associate a higher level of *unhu* with Christianity, and sometimes condemn Christians, where they are found wanting. This state of affairs might have been caused by the claims of superiority that Christianity makes.

Bibliography

Akrong, Abraham. "A Phenomenology of Witchcraft in Ghana." In *Imagining Evil: Witchcraft Beliefs and Accusations in Contemprary Africa,* edited by Gerrie ter Haar, 53–66. Trenton, NJ: Africa World, 2007.

Anderson, Allan. *Zion and Pentecost: The Spirituality and Experience of Pentecostal and Zionist/Apostolic Churches in South Africa.* Pretoria: University of South Africa Press, 2000.

Barrett, David B. *Schism and Renewal in Africa: An Analysis of Six Thousand Contemporary Religious Movements.* London: Oxford University Press, 1968.

Bhebe, Ngwabi. *Christianity and Traditional Religion in Western Zimbabwe 1859–1923.* London: Longman, 1979.

Bourdillon, M. F. C. *Religion and Society: A Text for Africa.* Gweru: Mambo, 1990.

———. *The Shona Peoples.* Gweru, Zimbabwe: Mambo, 1987.

Bucher, Hubert. *Spirits and Power: An Analysis of Shona Cosmology.* Cape Town: Oxford University Press, 1980.

Bullock, Charles. *Mashona Laws and Customs.* Salisbury, Zimbabwe: Argus, 1913.

———. *The Mashona (The Indigenous Natives of S. Rhodesia).* Westport, CT: Negro University Press, 1928.

Chavhunduka, Gordon. L. "Witchcraft and the Law in Zimbabwe." *Zambezia* VIII.ii (1980) 129–47.

Chigwedere, Aeneas S. *Lobola—The Pros and Cons.* Harare: Apex Holdings, 1982.

———. *From Mutapa to Rhodes: 1000 to 1890 A.D.* London: Macmillan, 1980.

Chikowero, Mhoze. *African Music, Power, and Being in Colonial Zimbabwe.* Indianapolis: Indiana University Press, 2015.

Chitakure, John. *The Pursuit of the Sacred: An Introduction to Religious Studies.* Eugene, OR: Wipf and Stock, 2016.

———. *Shona Women in Zimbabwe—A Purchased People? Marriage, Bridewealth, Domestic Violence, and Christian Traditions on Women.* AFRICS. Eugene, OR: Pickwick 2016.

Cox, Harvey. *Fire from Heaven: The Rise of Pentecostal Spirituality and the Reshaping of Religion in the Twenty-first Century.* New York: Addison-Wesley, 1995.

Crawford, J. R. *Witchcraft and Sorcery in Rhodesia.* London: Oxford University Press, 1967.

Creary, Nicholas M. *Domesticating a Religious Import: The Jesuits and the Inculturation of the Catholic Church in Zimbabwe, 1879–1980.* New York: Fordham University Press, 2011.

Daneel, M. L. *The God of the Matopos Hills: An Essay on the Mwari Cult in Rhodesia.* Leiden: Mouton, 1970.

———. *Old and New in Southern Shona Independent Churches, Vol. 1: Background and Rise of Major Movements.* Herderstraat 5. Leiden: Mouton, 1971.

———. *Quest for Belonging: An Introduction to a Study of African Independent Churches*. Gweru, Zimbabwe: Mambo, 1987.

———. *Zionism and Faith-Healing in Rhodesia: Aspects of an African Independent Church*. Leiden: Mouton, 1970.

Evans-Pritchard, E. E. *Witchcraft, Oracles, and Magic among the Azande*. New York: Oxford University Press, 1976.

Gelfand, Michael, ed. *The African Witch with Special Reference to Witchcraft Beliefs and Practice among the Shona of Rhodesia*. London: Livingstone, 1967.

———. *Gubulawayo and Beyond: Letters and Journals of the Early Jesuit Missionaries to the Zambesia (1879–1887)*. New York: Barnes and Noble, 1969.

———. *Shona Ritual with Special Reference to the Chaminuka Cult*. Cape Town: Juta, 1959.

———. *Shona Religion with Special Reference to the Makorekore*. Cape Town: Juta, 1962.

———. "UNHU—The Personality of the Shona." *Studies in Comparative Religion* 4.1 (1970). www.studiesincomparativereligion.com. Date accessed, 09/28/2016

Haffner, Paul. *The Sacramental Mystery*. Leominster, UK: Gracewing, 1999.

Idowu, E. Bolaji. *African Traditional Religion: A Definition*. Maryknoll, NY: Orbis, 1975.

Ikenga-Metuh, Emefie. *Comparative Studies of African Traditional Religions*. South Onitsha: IMICO, 1987.

Imasogie, O. *African Traditional Religion*. Ibadan, Nigeria: University Press, 1985, 52.

Kayode, J. O. *Understanding African Traditional Religion*. Ile-Ife, Nigeria: University of Ife Press, 1984.

Leclerc-Madlala, Suzanne. "Virginity Testing: Managing Sexuality in a Maturing HIV/AIDS Epidemic." In *Perspectives on Africa: A Reader in Culture, History, and Representation*, edited by Roy Richard Grinker, Stephen C. Lubkemann, and Christopher B. Steiner, 411–22. 2nd ed. Chichester, UK: Wiley-Blackwell, 2010.

Livingstone, David. *Missionary Travels and Researches in South Africa/ Journeys and Researches in South Africa*. Chapter 1. Presented to the Royal Geographic Society in London, 1952, and verified in 1857. Produced by Alan. R. Light and David Widger. Released on February 11, 2006 [EBook #1039], and updated on February 4, 2013: The Project Gutenberg EBook of Missionary Travels and Researches in South Africa, by David Livingstone; http://www.gutenberg.org/files/1039/1039-h/1039-h.htm#link2HCH0001, accessed on 10/22/2016.

Martin de Agar, Joseph T. *A Handbook on Canon Law*. 2nd ed. Rome: Wilson and Lafleur Ltee, 2007.

Maxwell, David. *African Gifts of the Spirit: The Rise of a Zimbabwean Transnational Religious Movement*. Athens, OH: Ohio University Press, 2006.

Mbiti, John S. *African Religions and Philosophy*. Oxford: Heinemann, 1990.

Mukonyora, Isabel. *Wandering a Gendered Wilderness: Suffering and Healing in an African Initiated Church*. New York: Lang, 2007.

Nasimiyu-Wasike, Anne, "Polygamy: A Feminist Critique." In *The Will to Arise: Women, Tradition, and the Church in Africa*, edited by Mercy Amba Oduyoye and Kanyoro, R. A. Musimbi, 101–18. 1992. Reprint. Eugene, OR: Wipf and Stock, 2005.

Nicolaides, A. "Early Portuguese Imperialism: Using the Jesuits in Mutapa Empire of Zimbabwe." *International Journal of Peace and Development Studies* 2.4 (2011) 132–37. http://www.academicjournals.org/IJPS. Accessed on 10/21/2016.

Oduyoye, Mercy Amba. *Beads and Strands: Reflections of an African Woman on Christianity in Africa*. Maryknoll, NY: Orbis, 2004.
———. *Daughters of Anowa: African Women and Patriarchy*. Maryknoll, NY: Orbis, 1995.
———. "Feminist Theology in an African Perspective." In *Paths of African Theology*, edited by Rosino Gibellini, 166–81. Maryknoll, NY: Orbis, 1994.
Opoku, Kofi Asare. *West African Traditional Religion*. Accra, Ghana: FEP, 1978.
Parrinder, Geoffrey. *African Traditional Religion*. Westport, CT: Greenwood, 1970.
———. *Witchcraft: European and African*. London: Faber and Faber, 1963.
Pindula. Website of the United Family International Church. http://www.pindula.co.zw/United_Family_International_Church, accessed on 10/27/2016.
Pope Francis. Apostolic Exhortation *Evangelii Gaudium*, Chapter 2, Section I, paragraph 69, November 24, 2013. http://w2.vatican.va/content/francesco/en/apost_exhortations/documents/papa-francesco_esortazione-ap_20131124_evangelii-gaudium.html#Challenges_to_inculturating_the_faith.
Presler, Titus Leonard. *Transfigured Night: Mission and Culture in Zimbabwe's Vigil Movement*. Pretoria: University of South Africa, 1999.
Quarcoopome, T. N. O. *West African Traditional Religion*. Ibadan, Nigeria: African Universities Press, 1987.
Ranger, Terence O. *The African Churches of Tanzania*. Dar es Salaam, Tanzania: East African, 1972.
———. *Voices from the Rocks: Nature, Culture, and History in the Matopos Hills of Zimbabwe*. Harare, Zimbabwe: Baobab, 1999.
Rayner, William. *The Tribe and Its Successors: An Account of African Traditional Life and European Settlement in Southern Rhodesia*. New York: Praeger, 1962.
Rodlach, Alexander. *Witches, Westerners, and HIV*. Walnut Creek, CA: Left Coast, 2006.
Schreiter, Robert. *Constructing Local Theologies*. Maryknoll, NY: Orbis, 1985.
———. *The New Catholicity: Theology between the Global and the Local*. Maryknoll. NY: Orbis, 2004.
Shaw, Carolyn Martin. *Women and Power in Zimbabwe: Promises of Feminism*. Urbana, IL: University of Illinois Press, 2015.
Shorter, Aylward. *African Culture and the Christian Church: An Introduction to Social and Pastoral Anthropology*. London: Chapman, 1973.
———. *Towards a Theology of Inculturation*. London: Chapman, 1988.
Sundkler, Bengt G. M. *Bantu Prophets in South Africa*. London: Oxford University Press, 1964.
Taylor, John V. *The Primal Vision: Christian Presence amid African Religion*. Philadelphia: Fortress, 1963.
Thomas, Lynn M. *Politics of the Womb: Women, Reproduction, and the State in Kenya*. Berkeley: University of California Press, 2003.
Thomas, Thomas Morgan. *Eleven Years in Central South Africa*. London: Snow, 1872.
Thorpe, S. A. *African Traditional Religions: An Introduction*. Pretoria: University of South Africa, 1992.
Turner, Harold W. *African Independent Church*. Oxford: Clarendon, 1967.
———. *History of an African Independent Church, Vols. 1–2: The Church of the Lord (Aladura)*. Oxford: Clarendon, 1967.
———. *Religious Innovation in Africa: Collected Essays on New Religious Movements*. Boston: Hall, 1979.

UFIC official webpage. http://www.ufiministries.org/index.php/features/about-ufi, accessed on 10/27/2016.
West, Martin. *Bishops and Prophets in a Black City.* Cape Town: Philip, 1975.
The Witchcraft Suppression Act (Chapter 73), 1899. http://www.parlzim.gov.zw/acts-list/witchcraft-suppression-act-9-19.
Zvobgo, C. J. M. *A History of Christian Missions in Zimbabwe 1890–1939.* Gweru, Zimbabwe: Mambo, 1996.

Index

Abenhla, 24n28
Abezanzi, 24n28
aborted fetus, avenging spirit of, 107
abstinence, sexual, 39, 193,
Achiuyu, 12, 13
activity, sexual, 33-34, 39-40, 48, 71, 92, 122, 195, 205-6
adultery, 57, 91, 95-96, 205
African Independent Churches, xi, 10, 34, 66-67, 98, 116, 127, 138, 147, 162-64, 167, 171, 188, 198
African Traditional Religion, xi, xiii, 3, 6, 7-10, 42, 68, 79, 148, 169-70, 186
Agar, Martin de, 67n37
Akrong, Abraham, 116n3, 135n23
Amahole, 24n28
Ancestor(s), xi, 3-5, 7-9, 14, 16, 23-25, 29, 32-33, 35-37, 40-41, 44, 48, 53-54, 56-58, 61-65, 68-69, 75, 77-83, 85-98, 102, 104, 113-14, 118, 121, 123, 140, 143, 146-47, 156, 158-59, 171, 190, 192, 205
Anderson, Allan, 174n31, 182n38
axis mundi, 37

barrenness, 56-59, 110, 117, 153-55, 175, 191, 196
Barrett, David B., 164n2, 171n26, 174n29
beast of motherhood, 53, 95, 101-2
bembera, 127-28, 157
Bhebe, Ngwabi, 23n25-24n29, 70n3-71n11
birth rites, 33
Bourdillon, M. F. C., 100n3, 132n15, 134n20, 117n4, 152n6, 154n7, 194

bride, 30, 48, 60, 95-96, 102, 211
bridewealth, 3-4, 30, 48-51, 53-57, 59, 66-67, 82, 92, 95, 102, 106-7, 189, 192, 194
British South Africa Company, xi, 8, 12, 27, 76, 115
Bucher, Hubert, 57, 73n16, 154n8, 167n15
bull, ancestral, 89
Bullock, Charles, 34n6, 35n8-36n12, 44, 56, 59n29-31, 70n5, 142n2

Caiado, Antonio, 12, 16
calamity, 95
catechists, 30, 173, 177, 182-83
Chavhunduka, Gordon. L., 115n1, 124
Chidavaenzi, Ignatius, 71
Chidziva Chepo, 73
Chigwedere, Aeneas S., 35n11, 41, 48n21, 53n26
Chikowero, Mhoze, 23, 29
chikwambo, 126
chimanda, 48
Chirazamauya, 75
chisinha, 144
Chitakure, John, 44n19, 49n22, 55, 148n1, 189n6, 195n16, 203
Christian(s), xii, 1, 5-11, 14, 19, 21-22, 27-30, 38, 62-63, 65-69, 76-78, 97-98, 111-13, 133, 137-38, 159-65, 167, 169-71, 178-81, 183-84, 190, 213
Christianity, xi, 2, 6-8, 10-12, 14-20, 22-23, 25, 27-28, 30, 38, 65, 67-69, 76-77, 97-98, 111-13, 136, 138, 146-47, 149, 151, 159-60, 162, 165, 168-69, 173, 182, 196-97, 210, 213

chronos, 26–27, 210
churches, Christian, xii, 8–10, 66, 97–98, 112–14, 116, 147, 160, 163, 168, 180, 197, 211–12
circumcision, 41–43, 66, 154, 189
cleansing ceremony, 63, 65, 68, 80–83, 85–86, 88, 89, 98, 140, 190–91
clitoridectomy, 66, 189, 196
concubines, 23, 174
Cox, Harvey, 167n18
Crawford, J. R., 127n11, 108n7, 131n13
Creary, Nicholas M., 17n9, 29n34, 68n38, 71n8, 76n18
Croonenburghs, Fr., 22
culture, 1, 2, 5–7, 21–22, 25, 30, 57, 61, 98, 145, 149, 160, 165, 171, 179–80, 186, 189, 197
culture, African, 30–31, 132, 149, 160, 171, 174, 181, 196
culture, European, 6–7, 21, 149, 196
culture, Shona, 16, 46, 57, 145, 202, 213

Daneel, M. L., 28n32, 71, 72n12, 73n14–15, 109, 165n6, 166–67, 171n25, 174n30, 175, 189n4
danga, 52–54, 56–57, 59
Danquah, J. B., 69
death rites, 61
Depelchin, Fr., 21–22
Divination, 141, 146–47, 153–54, 156
Divisi, 121–22
dual religiosity, 7, 30, 68
Dzivaguru, 73

Ethics, 199, 210–11
Ethiopia, 165–66
Ethiopian Churches, 165
Evans-Pritchard, E. E., 118, 128n12, 133n18, 152n5

filial respect, 202
First Chimurenga, 6

Gelfand, Michael, 3n3, 17n7, 21n19, 19, 50n23, 63n33, 71n10, 82, 96, 103n5, 143, 154n7, 155, 209n1
generosity, 1, 3, 10, 13, 105, 208
God, xi, 1–6, 9, 11, 13, 16, 19–24, 27, 29–30, 68–78, 82, 94, 97,
112–14, 116, 133, 137, 142, 147, 151–52, 159–60, 163, 166–68, 170–71, 173–74, 176–79, 181–84, 190, 197–98, 205
gratitude, xiii, 59, 208–9
grave, 61–64, 84–86, 106, 109–10, 117–19
greetings, 10, 199–201
Gupuro, 58–59
gwevedzi, 45–46

Hafner, Paul, 66n36
hakata, 154
harugwa, 90
healer, traditional, 14, 83, 86, 90, 127, 131, 134, 149
healing, 5, 42, 93, 98, 116, 132, 137–38, 141–43, 146–47, 152–56, 160, 162–62, 166, 168, 172, 174–76, 179–81, 183–84
heaven, xi, 1–1, 4–6, 8–9, 29, 68, 98, 113–14, 116, 212, 133
herbs, 29, 33, 36, 51, 57, 84, 93, 124, 142, 152–56, 159–60, 162
homilies, 168, 176–78
hosana, 72, 76

Idowu, E. B., 148n1
Ikenga-Metuh, Emefie, 83n5
Imasogie, O., 31, 61n32
immunizations, traditional, 38–40, 66
impotency, 59
incest, 3, 59, 82, 95–96, 121, 205–6, 211–12
inculturation, 30, 98, 180, 184

Jesuits, 2, 8, 17–23, 28, 77
Jesus Christ, 2, 7, 11, 18–19, 21, 25, 30, 97–98, 164–66, 168, 197

Kaguvi, Sekuru, 6
Kairos, 26–27
Karanga, xii, 50–51, 64, 66, 84, 90, 108, 118–20, 125, 142, 152, 158
Kayode, J. O., 91–92, 95n2
Kimbangu, Simon, 166
Kukumbira, 49
kurova guva, 29, 63–65, 68, 82, 85, 87–88, 96, 140

kutanda botso, 101, 103–4
kuzvarira, 188, 194

land, 3–4, 11, 14, 17–18, 23, 28, 70, 72–76, 90–93, 96, 104, 111, 121, 154, 159, 190
Leclerc-Madlala, Suzanne, 187n2, 193n12
lightning, 74–75, 125–26, 134
Livingstone, David, 151, 152n4, 159–60
Livingstonia Church, 171
Lobengula, King, 2, 12, 17–18, 25, 27–28, 100
London Missionary Society, 2, 8–9, 11, 17–76–77
longevity, 2, 4–5, 44, 56, 75, 81–82, 175, 180

Mabweadziva, 73
mainline churches, 10, 67, 98, 133, 138, 161–64, 169–70, 173–76, 180–85, 197–98
mamutsamurimo, 121, 143–44
mapositori, 138, 163
Mapunzaguta, Negomo, 12–17
marriage rites, 31, 44, 66,
marriage, 8, 30–32, 35, 43–44, 47–49, 51–58, 60, 66–67, 72, 80–81, 92, 98, 101–2, 104, 108, 132, 140, 144–45, 150, 184, 187–89, 191, 193–96, 198, 202–4, 209, 213
marriage, child, 184, 196, 198
marriage, polygamous, 22–23, 67
masungiro, 34–35
Matonjeni, 5, 9, 20, 68, 70, 72–78, 113, 142
Matopos Hills, xi, 1, 9, 70–71, 76, 78, 171
Maxwell, David, 166n11
mazioni, 138, 163
Mbiti, J. S., 33n4, 69, 80
mbonga, 72, 76–77
Medical Practitioners, Traditional, xi, 3–5, 10, 94, 109, 117–18, 121, 125–27, 131–32, 137–38, 144, 146–48, 150, 152–54, 156–57, 159–60, 162, 171–72, 175

mermaid, 153
Messianic, 164, 166
missionaries, 1–2, 4–9, 11–12, 16, 18–30, 65, 67–70, 76–78, 97–98, 111–12, 115, 137, 146–47, 150, 159, 171–74, 190, 197, 211
missionaries, Christian, 1–2, 4, 6, 8, 10–11, 65, 69–71, 77, 97, 111, 113, 136
Mlingo, Emmanuel, 161
Moffat, John S., 17, 24
Moffat, Robert, 17
morality, 91, 124, 165, 194, 199, 210–12
mother-in-law, 50, 53–54, 60, 102, 200, 202–3, 211
mubobobo, 122
Mukonyora, Isabel, 189n5, 192, 196
munyayi, 49, 53
mupfuwira, 122–23
muposo, 125, 141
muroora, 55, 60
murundu, 42
Musikavanhu, 74, 77
Musiki, 73, 77
Muslims, 15, 41–42
Mutapa Palace/Court, 12–13, 15–16,
Mutapa State (Empire), 2, 8, 12, 14–15, 16–17, 41
Mutemwa Shrine, 181
Muyambi, Lazarus, Fr., 161
Mwari, 9, 20, 23, 70–73, 75–78, 94, 142, 171
Mwedzi Myth, 73–74
Mzilikazi, King, 2, 12, 17

n'anga, 134, 152–62
Nasimiyu-Wasike, Anne, 190n7, 191
Ndebele, xi, 8, 11, 17–28, 70, 74, 99–100, 142–43
nduma, 47
Nehanda, Mbuya, 6, 195
ngomwa, 57
Ngozi, 9, 100–1, 106–11, 113–14, 141, 157, 188–89
Nicolaides, A., 13
non-violence, 209
Nyadenga, 74

Oduyoye, Mercy A., 187, 191, 197–98
Opoku, Kofi A., 82n3, 83n6, 91n7

Parrinder, Geoffrey, 33n5, 43n18, 69n1, 117, 119, 131n14, 136n24, 149, 150n3
placenta, 36, 41, 65
poisoning, 124
polygamy, 22–23, 29, 30, 67, 98, 133, 171, 174, 184, 190, 195, 197–98, 213
Pope Francis, 176, 179, 180n36, 198
Portuguese, 12, 13, 15–16, 143,
Presler, Titus L., 169
Prestage, Peter, Fr., 18, 22, 28
Priest, 9, 11–16, 21–22, 29, 65–66, 68, 71–72, 75–78, 113, 169, 176–79, 182,
Priest, Roman Catholic, 176–79
prophets, 38, 78, 138, 147, 162, 175–76, 181
Prosperity, 2–3, 5, 20, 75, 168, 174, 180–81
puberty rites, 41

Quarcoopome, T. N. O., 33n2, 118n7, 133n16

rain doctor, 151, 159–60
rainmaking, 76, 142, 159
Ranger, Terence O., 23, 172n27, 173n28
rape, 192, 206, 212
Rayner, William, 13n2, 33n3, 99, 141n1, 142n3, 146n6
Rhodes, Cecil J., xi, 1, 23, 28, 71, 76
rites of passage, xi, 4–5, 8, 31, 40, 65–67, 98
ritual, 2, 4–5, 7–10, 29–43, 53–56, 58, 61–68, 74–75, 77–78, 80–81, 83–90, 93–98, 101, 103–4, 106–9, 114, 121–22, 130, 141–45, 150–52, 157–61, 166, 170, 179, 183, 189–92, 195, 205
Rodlach, Alexander, 123n9
Roman Catholic Church, xi, 7, 9–10, 19, 30, 66–68, 98, 138, 161, 163–64, 170, 176, 178–83, 185, 197–98, 211–12

rugaba, 49, 51–52
ruhahu, 63, 84, 106–7
rukwa, 123–24, 136

Samasimba, 75, 77
Schreiter, Robert, 7
sex, 24, 33–35, 40, 119, 122, 175, 187–88, 192–93, 195, 204–6
seximania, 39
sexuality, 10, 43, 188,
shavi, 10, 63, 140–47, 157–58
Shaw, Carolyn M., 188, 194n14
Shorter, Aylward, 2n2, 5n4, 134n19–21, 139
Silveira, Gonzalo da, Fr., 2, 8, 11–17
son-in-law, 46, 49–53, 56–57, 59, 95, 102, 106–7, 191, 200, 202, 211
spirits, Alien, 3–4, 10, 140–43, 145–46, 152, 158
spirits, avenging, 9, 54, 61, 83, 96, 99–105, 108–14, 157, 188–89, 196, 207–8
spirits, evil, 3–4, 8, 33–34, 37–38, 65–66, 83, 86, 91, 104, 127, 138, 141, 158, 161, 167, 172, 175, 179,
suicide, 83, 110–11
Sundkler, Bengt G. M., 165–67, 170, 171n23
Sykes, William, 17
syncretism, 7

Taylor, John V., 1
telepathy, 133
Thomas, Lynn M., 194n13
Thomas, Thomas M., 17, 20–21, 76
Thorpe, S. A., 70n4
totem, 40–41, 54, 58, 84, 101, 155, 189, 203
Tsikamutanda, 127, 156
Turner, Harold W., 164–165, 167n13
Typology, 10, 164–65, 167

UFIC, 167–68
Umbilical code, 37–38, 41, 89–90, 93, 96,
Unhu, 2–3, 82, 199, 201–13
Urayai, Augustine, Fr., 161

VaRemba, 41–42
vatezvara, 50–54
virginity, 48, 66, 187–88, 192–93, 204, 212

West, Martin, 167, 175
widow, 87–88, 168, 190, 195,
wife, *ngozi* of, 108, 113, 188–89
witch(es), 3–5, 9, 15–16, 24–25, 36–38, 47, 62–63, 65, 83–84, 102, 108–9, 115–39, 141, 143–44, 147, 149–50, 156–59, 171–72, 191, 197, 201,
Witchcraft Suppression Act, (Chapter 73, 1899), 115, 137, 146, 157

witchcraft, xi, 5, 9–10, 24–25, 47, 76, 83, 98, 102, 108, 115–17, 119–39, 141, 143–44, 147, 150, 156–57, 164, 172, 180, 191, 196–97, 208
witch-doctor, 5, 149–50, 152, 159

Zhezha, Mai, 141, 144–45, 160
ZINATHA, 162
Zionist Churches, 165–66
zumbani, 155
Zvibinge, 50–51
zvidhoma, 119–20, 132
Zvobgo, C. J. M., 22

www.ingramcontent.com/pod-product-compliance
Lightning Source LLC
Chambersburg PA
CBHW051640230426
43669CB00013B/2385